International guidelines for estimating the costs of substance abuse

Second edition

Eric Single, David Collins, Brian Easton, Henrick Harwood, Helen Lapsley, Pierre Kopp and Ernesto Wilson

WHO Library Cataloguing-in-Publication Data

International guidelines for estimating the costs of substance abuse /
Eric Single ... [et al.].

1.Substance abuse - economics 2.Substance-related disorders - economics
3.Costs and cost analysis 4.Guidelines I.Single, Eric. II.International
Symposium on Estimating the Economic and Social Costs of Substance Abuse
(3rd : 2000 : Alberta, Canada). Working Group.

ISBN 92 4 154582 8 (LC/NLM classification: HV 4998)

© World Health Organization 2003

All rights reserved. Publications of the World Health Organization can be obtained from Marketing and Dissemination, World Health Organization, 20 Avenue Appia, 1211 Geneva 27, Switzerland (tel: +41 22 791 2476; fax: +41 22 791 4857; email: bookorders@who.int). Requests for permission to reproduce or translate WHO publications – whether for sale or for noncommercial distribution – should be addressed to Publications, at the above address (fax: +41 22 791 4806; email: permissions@who.int).

The designations employed and the presentation of the material in this publication do not imply the expression of any opinion whatsoever on the part of the World Health Organization concerning the legal status of any country, territory, city or area or of its authorities, or concerning the delimitation of its frontiers or boundaries. Dotted lines on maps represent approximate border lines for which there may not yet be full agreement.

The mention of specific companies or of certain manufacturers' products does not imply that they are endorsed or recommended by the World Health Organization in preference to others of a similar nature that are not mentioned. Errors and omissions excepted, the names of proprietary products are distinguished by initial capital letters.

The World Health Organization does not warrant that the information contained in this publication is complete and correct and shall not be liable for any damages incurred as a result of its use.

The named authors alone are responsible for the views expressed in this publication.

Printed in Switzerland

Contents

Acknowledgements	v
Executive summary	vi
1. Estimating the costs of substance abuse: introduction	**1**
1.1 Introduction	2
1.2 The purposes of economic cost estimates	2
1.3 Organization of this report	3
2. A layperson's guide to economic cost estimation	**5**
2.1 Introduction	6
2.2 Economic cost studies	6
2.2.1 Economic cost studies: a type of COI study	6
2.2.2 Costs to whom?	7
2.2.3 What constitutes a cost – social vs. private costs	8
2.2.4 Further costs: productivity losses	11
2.2.5 The ultimate cost: placing a value on life itself	11
2.3 Demographic approach vs. the human capital approach	12
2.4 Prevalence vs. incidence based approaches	13
2.5 What economic cost studies are not	13
2.6 Interpretation of substance abuse cost estimates	15
3. Some theoretical issues in the application of the framework	**17**
3.1 Definition and measurement of abuse	18
3.2 Definition of costs	18
3.3 Treatment and measurement of addictive consumption	19
3.4 Human capital and demographic approaches	20
3.5 Choice of appropriate discount rates	20
3.6 Treatment of private costs and benefits	21
3.7 Treatment and measurement of intangible costs, including willingness-to-pay	21
3.8 Comparing and presenting estimates of the value of human life	22
3.9 The positive economic impact of consumption	23
3.10 Estimation of avoidable costs	24
3.11 Prevalence vs. incidence based estimates	24
3.12 Crime and substance abuse	25
3.13 Who bears the social costs of substance abuse?	27

3.14 The budgetary impact of substance abuse	27
3.15 Special considerations in drug-producing countries	29

4. Towards a common framework: the matrix of costs and issues of measurement — 31

4.1 Which substances to study	32
4.2 Major types of costs included in cost estimation studies	33
4.3 Health care and health services	36
4.3.1 Treatment for substance abuse	36
4.3.2 Health treatment for co-morbidity and trauma	37
4.4 Productivity costs	38
4.4.1 Premature mortality	38
4.4.2 Morbidity – lost employment or productivity	39
4.4.3 Treatment of non-workforce mortality and morbidity	40
4.5 Crime and law enforcement costs	42
4.5.1 Criminal justice expenditures	42
4.5.2 Crime victim's time losses	42
4.5.3 Incarceration	43
4.5.4 Crime career costs	43
4.6 Other costs	44
4.6.1 Treatment of research, education and law enforcement costs	44
4.6.2 Prevention and other public health efforts	44
4.6.3 Property destruction for crime or accidents	44
4.6.4 Welfare costs	45

5. Data requirements and special considerations for developing countries — 47

5.1 Data requirements for estimating social costs	48
5.2 Closing the data gaps	49

6. Interpretation of cost estimates and the relevance to evaluation of policies and programmes — 51

Summary and conclusions — 56

Appendix A–Glossary of common terms used on economic cost studies — 57

Appendix B– The evaluation of economies with significant drug production industries — 65

Appendix C–Comparing the social costs of substance abuse to GDP — 71

Appendix D—Application of the guidelines in cost estimation studies — 75

References — 77

Endnotes — 80

Acknowledgements

This document derives from a series of on-going symposia organized by the Canadian Centre on Substance Abuse (CCSA) with the support of a variety of regional, national and international organisations. The First International Symposium on Estimating the Social and Economic Costs of Substance Abuse was held in Banff, Alberta, in 1994, and the Second International Symposium on Estimating the Social and Economic Costs of Substance Abuse was held in Montibello, Quebec, in 1995. The first symposium focused on issues of economic modeling while the second symposium focused on epidemiological issues involved in estimating deaths, hospitalizations and crime attributable to substance abuse. These meetings were organized and co-hosted by the CCSA with funding support from the following organisations: the Alcohol Advisory Council of New Zealand; the Addiction Centre, Foothills Medical Centre, Canada; the Alberta Alcoholism and Drug Abuse Commission; the Australian Department of Human Services and Health; Canada's Drug Strategy Secretariat of Health Canada; the Center for Substance Abuse Prevention, USA; the Foothills Hospital Foundation, Canada; The Friends of Matt Newell Fund, Canada; the Health Promotion Directorate, Alcohol and Other Drugs Programs, Health Canada; the International Labour Organization, Switzerland; the National Institute on Drug Abuse, USA. The financial support of these organizations and the expertise that individual participants brought to the meetings are gratefully acknowledged.

The first edition of the guidelines was developed by a working group designated by participants at these meetings, consisting of Eric Single (Canada, chair), David Collins (Australia), Brian Easton (New Zealand), Henrick Harwood (USA), Helen Lapsley (Australia) and Alan Maynard (UK). The guidelines were published by the CCSA in 1996, and provided the basis for further cost estimation studies in Australia (Collins and Lapsley, 1995), Canada (Single et al., 1998) and the US (Harwood et al., 1999). The first edition of the guidelines have also been available at the CCSA website (http://www.ccsa.ca), and were used in a number of other cost estimation studies in Europe and South America.

The Third International Symposium on Estimating the Social and Economic Costs of Substance Abuse, held in Banff, Canada in the fall of 2000, focused on emerging issues in the application of the guidelines, particularly their utility in developing economies and in drug-producing countries. It was decided that a second edition of the guidelines should be prepared and an expanded working group was struck, consisting of Eric Single (Canada, chair), David Collins (Australia), Brian Easton (New Zealand), Henrick Harwood (USA), Helen Lapsley (Australia), Pierre Kopp (France) and Ernesto Wilson (Colombia). The group held a 3-day working meeting in Washington, D.C., in May of 2001 at the offices of the Inter-American Agency on Narcotic Drugs (CICAD) and finalised this second edition of the guidelines.

As with the original guidelines, this second edition of the guidelines is truly a collaborative effort. The organisation and first sections of these guidelines are based in large measure on planning documents prepared by Eric Single. Section 2, "A Layperson's Guide to the Evaluation of Social and Economic Costs of Substance Abuse", was prepared by Brian Easton. The description of a common framework for economic cost studies in Section 3 draws upon material from presentations at the three symposia, and particularly the paper at the first symposium by Henrick Harwood entitled "Selected Issues and Parameters In the Design and Performance of Cost-of-illness Studies for Substance Abuse". David Collins, Brian Easton, Helen Lapsley, Pierre Kopp and Eric Single also made significant contributions to the discussion of issues in Section 3. The detailed discussion in Section 4 of the issues involved in the application of this framework, which also draws upon the background papers, is based in part on a working paper by David Collins and Helen Lapsley entitled "Technical Issues in Abuse Cost Estimation". Parts of this discussion were also prepared by Brian Easton, Henrick Harwood and Eric Single. Ernesto Wilson, David Collins, Helen Lapsley and Eric Single contributed to the development of Section 5 on data requirements in developing economies. The concluding sections of these guidelines represent a collaboration of all members of the Working Group. Appendix A, the "Glossary of common terms used on economic cost studies", was prepared by Brian Easton and Robert Bowie. Brian Easton also drafted Appendix B and Appendix C with significant input from all of the members of the working group. Eric Single was responsible for pulling the various components together and editing the final text.

Special mention should be made of Jacques LeCavalier for the central role he played in coordinating and organizing the three symposia, and for his enthusiastic promotion of the development of these guidelines.

Finally, thanks are due to Maristela Monteiro, Coordinator, and Isidore Obot, Scientist, Management of Substance Dependence, Department of Mental Health and Substance Dependence, World Health Organization, for their roles in the finalization and publication of this document.

Executive Summary

The use of alcohol, tobacco, pharmaceuticals and illicit drugs involves a wide variety of adverse health and social consequences. There is a strong need for improved estimates of the economic costs of substance abuse. Cost estimates help to prioritize substance abuse issues, provide useful information for targeting programming, and identify information gaps. The development of improved cost estimates also offers the potential to develop more complete cost-benefit analyses of policies and programmes aimed at reducing the harm associated with the use of psychoactive substances.

This document presents a general framework for the development of cost estimates. Studies of the economic costs of substance abuse are described as a type of cost-of-illness study in which the impact of substance abuse on the material welfare of a society is estimated by examining the social costs of treatment, prevention, research, law enforcement and lost productivity plus some measure of the quality of life years lost, relative to a counterfactual scenario in which there is no substance abuse.

A matrix of the types of costs to be considered is presented, and there is a detailed discussion of the theoretical issues involved, including: the definition of abuse, determination of causality, comparison of the demographic and human capital approaches to cost estimation, the treatment and measurement of addictive consumption, the treatment of private costs, the measurement of intangible costs, the treatment of non-workforce mortality and morbidity, the treatment of research, education, law enforcement costs, the estimation of avoidable costs and budgetary impact of substance abuse.

Special considerations are discussed with regard to developing economies and drug-producing countries. The guidelines conclude with a brief discussion of future directions, with particular attention to the expansion of economic cost studies to developing countries, and the implications of these guidelines to research agendas and data collection systems.

Estimating the costs of substance abuse: introduction

1.1 Introduction

There is a strong interest in many countries regarding the development of scientifically valid, credible estimates of the economic costs of drugs, alcohol and tobacco. The costs of substance abuse represent an issue of key interest to stakeholders, policy makers and the media. Knowledge of the costs of resources associated with alcohol, tobacco and drug abuse informs decisions related to funding and to interventions, which are designed to reduce abuse. Relatively few countries have attempted to estimate the costs of substance abuse. Such estimates are fraught with methodological difficulties resulting in widely varying estimates.

In May 1994 an international symposium was held in Banff, Canada, to discuss the issues involved in estimating the social and economic costs of substance abuse, and to seek a consensus on the most appropriate model. The purpose of the meeting was to explore the feasibility of establishing an internationally acceptable common methodology for estimating the costs of alcohol and other drugs. The symposium in Banff brought together persons with experience and expertise in dealing with the issues of costs estimation. Three papers were presented reviewing the current state of knowledge and exploring various methodological issues.[1]

There was a general agreement that it is possible and desirable to develop a set of guidelines regarding the estimation of the costs of substance use and abuse. The participants at the Banff symposium also agreed that the guidelines should be viewed as only the first step towards the development of improved and more internationally comparable estimates of the social and economic costs of substance use and abuse. A working committee consisting of the Eric Single, David Collins, Brian Easton, Henrick Harwood, Helen Lapsley and Alan Maynard drafted the first set of guidelines that were subsequently published by the Canadian Centre on Substance Abuse.

In 1995 a second symposium on estimating the economic costs of substance abuse was held in Montebello, Quebec. Whereas the first symposium had focused on modeling and methodological issues, this symposium focused more on epidemiological and practical issues involved in deriving cost estimates. In 2000 a third symposium was held in Banff, Alberta. This symposium focused on the results of cost studies using the guidelines, as well as special considerations involved in conducting cost estimation studies in developing economies and in drug-producing countries. It was decided to expand the working group to include economists from Europe (Pierre Kopp) and from South America (Ernesto Wilson). Following a special meeting at the offices of the Inter-American Agency on Narcotic Drugs (CICAD) in Washington in May, 2001, the following revised guidelines have been prepared.

1.2 The purposes of economic cost estimates

The need for estimates of the economic costs of substance abuse is almost self-evident. It is well established that the use of alcohol, tobacco and other drugs involves a large number of adverse health and social consequences. Thus, in most countries there are national policies for substance abuse, unlike for most other commodities. Because the justification for special regulation is the economic and social costs, and also because economic policy instruments are used in the regulation of these substances, it makes good sense to have sound estimates of the costs of substance abuse.

Estimates of the social and economic costs of substance abuse serve many purposes. First, economic cost estimates are frequently used to argue that policies on alcohol, tobacco and other drugs should be given a high priority on the public policy agenda. The public is entitled to a quality standard against which individual cost estimation studies can be assessed. Without such a standard there will be a tendency by the advocates for each social problem to overbid, adding in additional items to make their concern a suitably high (even exaggerated) number.

Second, cost estimates help to appropriately target specific problems and policies. It is important to know which psychoactive substances involve the greatest economic costs. For example, the recent study by Collins and Lapsley[2] concluded that the costs of alcohol and tobacco far exceeds the social costs from illicit drugs in Australia, thus focusing greater attention on public policy towards the licit drugs. Would a similar conclusion be reached in other countries? The specific types of cost may also draw our attention to specific areas which need public attention, or where specific measures may be effective.

Third, economic cost studies help to identify information gaps, research needs and desirable refinements to national statistical reporting systems. Indeed, it will be argued in this report that the development of improved, internationally comparable methods for estimating the costs of substance abuse should be attempted, insofar as possible, within the framework of the existing System of National Accounts (SNA). This system, which is best known for the Gross Domestic Product (GDP) measure[3] of total market activity, is oriented towards production and market activities, and does not generally cover important activities which occur outside the market, or affect the quality of life, and death. Hopefully, national accounting systems could be expanded and modified to facilitate economic cost studies, which are concerned with non-market activities and mortality. The development of estimates of the costs of substance abuse in the framework of the System of National Accounts would be a further step in the improvement and refinement of national accounting systems, increasing their relevance and usefulness.

Last but not least, the development of improved estimates of the costs of substance abuse offers the potential to provide baseline measures to determine the efficacy of drug policies and programmes intended to reduce the damaging consequences of alcohol, tobacco and other drug use. Estimates of the social costs can assist policy makers in evaluating outcomes, as expressed in terms of changes in social costs in constant dollar terms. Estimates of social costs can also facilitate cross-national comparisons of the consequences of substance abuse and different approaches to confronting those consequences. Are the costs of alcohol consumption higher in less restrictive societies? Are the social costs of cannabis greater in countries where it has been decriminalised? Other things being equal, is there less drug abuse in countries where a greater proportion of the costs are borne by the individual? Ultimately, cost estimates could be used to construct social cost functions for optimal tax policy and national target setting.

Perhaps most immediately promising is the prospect for cost estimates to be extended to more comprehensive cost-benefit analyses of specific drug policies and programmes. Without a national (and preferably international) standard, individual analyses are of limited utility, because the results are not comparable, and their conclusions can easily become dependent upon idiosyncratic assumptions which the analyst has to invent.

1.3 Organization of this report

The following document presents the second edition of a set of international guidelines on estimating the social and economic costs of substance. These guidelines are subject to further revision and refinement as we develop greater experience and improved databases. The guidelines begin with a description of economic cost studies oriented toward non-economists. A detailed glossary of terms is attached as Appendix A.

Section 3 presents a framework for the development of cost estimates. The major principle underlying the decision regarding which costs to include is the robustness of the estimates, which is in turn dependent on the availability of data. The matrix of factors to consider is generally limited to costs. It is recommended that data on benefits be collected wherever possible, and the revenue benefits are included in the calculation of budgetary impact, discussed in the next section.

Section 4 discusses conceptual and methodological issues in the application of this framework. The purpose is not to advocate a particular approach, but to describe alternatives and discuss the advantages and disadvantages of each approach for particular purposes. The following issues are discussed:

- definition and measurement of abuse
- definition of costs
- focus on adverse consequences rather than consumption per se

- causality
- the demographic and human capital approaches to cost estimation
- treatment and measurement of addictive consumption
- treatment of private costs and benefits
- treatment and measurement of intangibles
- treatment of non-workforce mortality and morbidity
- treatment of research, education, law enforcement costs
- estimation of avoidable costs
- estimation of budgetary impact: costs and benefits to include

Section 5 discusses special considerations for developing countries, outlining the key data requirements and prospects for closing data gaps. In Section 6, the interpretation of results is discussed, as well as the relevance of cost estimates to policy and programme development. The guidelines conclude in Section 7 with a brief discussion of future directions, with particular attention to the implications of these guidelines to research agendas and data collection systems.

These guidelines provide a framework rather than a rigorous methodology to be applied in every situation. It is recognized that there will not be sufficient data in many countries to implement the recommendations in this document. However, in many countries it will be possible to develop reasonable estimates for some, if not most, of the costs associated with substance abuse. It is hoped that these guidelines will help facilitate the development of more economic cost studies and enhance the comparability of such estimates. Although a manual providing detailed instructions on how to conduct cost estimation studies may be developed in the future, the following guidelines should be viewed as a general theoretical and methodological framework for such studies. The application of the guidelines in cost estimation studies is discussed in Appendix D.

The guidelines are only a tentative first step in a process aimed at developing more reliable and credible estimates of the costs of substance abuse. The next step in this process will be to apply the recommended procedures in new national and regional studies. This in turn should lead to further refinements to these guidelines. The long-term goal is to move from cost estimation to cost effectiveness analyses, and eventually to cost-benefit analyses of substance abuse policies and programmes.

A layperson's guide to economic cost estimation

2.1 Introduction

Like other professions, economists rely on a substantial body of common understanding, which they assume in their professional communications. As a consequence, non-economists can be confused by the writings and conversations of economists, even though these communications may be perfectly intelligible within the profession. This problem of communication with outsiders is especially unfortunate where the issue involves other professions, as is the case in the multidisciplinary field of substance abuse.

Thus it is appropriate to begin the discussion of economic cost studies by elaborating for the non-economist the implicit assumptions that the economists use. Simplification has been necessary, which means that some of the subtlety of the professional discourse may be lost. Obviously then, this discussion cannot cover all the points in the guidelines, nor does it superseded them. But hopefully it will enable those from other professions involved with substance abuse to have a better insight into the issues which trouble economists.

The discussion in this section is organized around three interrelated topics: what economic cost studies are, what different approaches may be taken to estimating economic costs and what economic cost studies are not.

2.2 Economic cost studies

In brief, the study of the economic costs of problems associated with the use of psychoactive substances is (1) a type of cost-of-illness study (2) in which the impact of substance abuse on the material welfare of a society is estimated by examining (3) the *social costs* of resources expended for treatment, prevention, research and law enforcement, plus (4) losses of production due to increased morbidity and mortality, plus (5) some measure for the quality of life years lost, relative to a counterfactual scenario in which there is no substance abuse. Each part of this statement bears elaboration.

2.2.1 Economic cost studies: a type of cost-of-illness (COI) study

The evaluation of the economic and social costs of substance abuse belongs to the genre of cost-of-illness studies (COI). Superficially a COI study involves combining an epidemiological database with financial information to generate an amount valued in monetary terms which purports to say something about the costs to society of a particular disease. Typically the magnitude is large, or large enough, to be used to draw attention to the condition as one to which policy makers, research funders, and researchers, ought to pay attention.

It will be clear from the intensity in which economists debate each calculation, that they have in mind some conceptual framework. The total is not just some gee-whiz figure designed to give a significant place to this or that illness in the public debate. So what are economists think they are doing? Moreover, why do they disagree?

At the heart of the economist's approach is that all relevant costs are *opportunity costs*, as it is the case when an activity (such as an illness) prevents resources being used for some other purpose, and so an opportunity is forgone. Thus COI studies rest on the proposition that if the illness were not to exist, then the resources that a society uses for treatment and other related purposes could be deployed in some other way.

Sitting behind the opportunity cost is *a counterfactual scenario*, that is, a description of an alternative state of affairs, by which the opportunity cost would be assessed. Often the counterfactual proposition is not controversial. For instance we might assume in a COI study of some viral infection, that the alternative scenario was no viral infection.

In the substance abuse field the alternative can be more arguable. For instance, the counterfactual to a situation of alcohol abuse might be that the abusers switch their consumption to mineral water and other health enhancing commodities, or it might be that abusers switch their consumption to narcotics. The latter is an extreme example, and usually a COI study assumes a switch to nondamaging activities, but sometimes the specific counterfactual situation is unclear.

Apart from disputes over the most appropriate counterfactual proposition, there are also disagreements that arise over what should or should not be included as a cost, as well as how that cost is to be valued or measured. These differences do not arise because of different underlying fundamental frameworks, but because the common framework has been applied in different ways, so practical considerations have led to the treatment of the same issue in different ways.

This is true for COI studies. The fundamental framework is "value theory", the role and interpretation of market price, which has been developed rigorously over the post-war period. Two practical applications of that theory are (1) in the *System of National Accounts* (SNA) and (2) *cost-benefit analysis* (CBA), which is a method of evaluation of alternative actions or treatments.

An integral assumption of value theory is that consumers value their own consumption, and that they rationally seek to maximize the value of their consumption as best they can, subject to various limitations such as their income and borrowing power. Thus, it is assumed that when a person buys a potato, a beer or an illicit drug, the cost of the purchase is offset by the benefits the consumer obtains from its use. Many who are knowledgeable about alcohol, tobacco and drug dependence would challenge the veracity of this assumption. Addictive behaviour seems to violate the assumption of rational consumer behaviour. How then is the economic analysis to deal with this situation?

One approach is to treat the psychoactive substances as conventional commodities, assuming that even dependent users are consuming rationally, according to their lights if not that of wiser counsel. In this case the perceived benefits of consumption exceed the outlay on the substance, and the transaction is treated as rational, just as purchases of other commodities, such as potatoes.

Collins and Lapsley[4] offer another approach, which attempts to modify the assumption of rational consumer behaviour in value theory, without destroying the entire paradigm. They estimate a proportion of drug consumption which is judged to be excessive. For that portion of consumption, they treat drug expenditure by users as zero under the counterfactual scenario in which there is no drug abuse, on the basis that dependent users receive no benefit from use. (Indeed, many users wish they had never taken up drug use.) This permits them to count expenditures on drugs by dependent users as a cost in the current actual scenario. This is a plausible alternative, which does not undermine value theory, although it leaves the difficult task of determining what proportion of substance use is dependent use.

The problem of how to resolve addictive consumption with the assumption of rational consumer behaviour is not fully resolved. The key point for the non-economist is that a main objective of the economist's approach in economic cost studies is to retain the well-established value theory paradigm, but to adapt it for the consumer behaviour which addiction implies.

2.2.2 Costs to whom? – cost studies in the System of National Accounts framework

Newspaper stories often cite "costs" of various social problems or negative events, such as the loss of a business convention, the impact of poor weather on tourism or the dire economic consequences of a professional sports strike. Frequently, such estimates lack credibility, as costs are magnified by following the flow of dollars from one party to the next, with little or no consideration of alternative uses for the money. For example, the money spent by a tourist or baseball fan at a restaurant is counted, then the money spent by the restaurant to food wholesalers, then the farmer's income, as well as income and other taxes paid by workers at each stage, and so forth. The fact that the money spent by local residents could have been used for alternative purposes is not considered. It is not surprising that cost figures such as these are viewed with scepticism. A cost for one person is typically a benefit to another. To the business manager who no longer has to pay for his or her staff to attend the cancelled conference, to the potential tourists who stayed at home and to the baseball fan whose game was cancelled by a strike, the "costs" of these cancelled events are really savings.

In short, to be credible, estimates of the costs of substance abuse must be clear with regard to what constitutes a cost, who bears these costs, and the boundaries which should be placed on the economic ramifications of negative impacts.

Cost-of-illness studies are quite precise in this regard: they estimate the impact of illness on a measure of material welfare in a society, closely related to the Gross Domestic Product. The GDP is generated in the System of National Accounts (SNA) by combining expenditure and production data with accounting information to produce an aggregate statistic valued in monetary terms. The Gross Domestic Product is not an arbitrary set of decisions about what is to be included and how each item is to be valued. Rather the aim is to encompass all market transactions valuing them at their marginal private value (or utility), which is usually equal to the market price (including indirect taxes). An increase of so many monetary units in the GDP can be interpreted as an increase in the sum of consumer utility of the same amount of monetary units.

In order to appreciate the significance of COI estimates in this framework, consider the counterfactual situation where people choose not to eat potatoes, but switch their expenditure to other products (say pasta). Clearly there will be a disruption among potato producers, but this will be offset by an expansion of pasta production. We take these two effects as (largely) balancing out, in which case there will be no change in GDP, even though there is a change in the composition of GDP.

What, we might ask, is the cost-of-potatoes to the economy? An answer might be that it is the cost of production and distribution. However, this is offset by the benefits to consumers of eating potatoes. More formally, we see that in the counterfactual situation, where there are no potatoes (but there is more pasta), there is no change to GDP. So we assess the social cost-of-potatoes to be zero. Note that we are not here assuming that the cost of potatoes is zero to consumers. They are a real cost to them but it is assumed to be offset by the benefits to them of the potatoes, and which is taken into account when they make the (private) decision to buy them.

2.2.3 What constitutes a cost? – social vs. private costs

Thus, where the costs of a commodity are largely limited to private costs, the economic impact is estimated at approximately zero. None of this should appear extraordinary. What is unusual is when we consider the same situation as it applies to psychoactive substances, which carries *social costs* as well as private costs.

To simplify, we shall illustrate the argument with tobacco, because it is probably the simplest of all the drugs, and its economic impact is the most transparent.[5] This time our counterfactual scenario is that there is no tobacco consumption, and there has been none in the past, so that smokers switch their consumption to some standard commodities (such as potatoes). In effect we are assuming that tobacco was never introduced to the society under consideration, and that potential smokers did not choose another drug (such as cannabis).

At first it might appear that this story was no different from the one about potatoes. But tobacco generates ill health, which requires medical care. The lack of smoking would mean that a significant quantity of medical resources would no longer be needed for the care of smoking induced sickness, and could be used for some other purposes. (It would also result in other savings, such as the cost of cleaning up litter and the costs of smoking-related fires.) The counterfactual is a little vague on what exactly is the alternative, but in the context it is not likely to matter. What is critical here is that we have a resource use consequent on the smoking, which is not being offset by some benefit to smokers when they decided to smoke.

The terminology that is being used here may differ somewhat from that used in some of the economic literature on the subject. In normal economic terminology, social costs generally equal private decision costs plus external costs. Private decision costs refer to the costs taken into account by the individuals making consumption decisions. (We use the term private decision costs here rather than simply private costs to avoid confusion with the distinction between private vs. public costs.) External costs (or externalities) refer to those costs that are external to the individual making the consumption decision, such as the costs that smoking causes to non-smokers. The inclusion of such externalities as part of social costs is uncontroversial. Indeed, external costs generally constitute virtually all of the total social costs in economic analyses because private decision costs are usually offset by private benefits. In the case of substance abuse, however, the situation is complicated by the fact that much of the private decision costs involves addictive consumption where the assumption that there are offsetting private benefits is subject to question. In addition to the consumers bearing the cost of the consumption decision themselves, a private decision cost must generally involve a rational decision by a fully informed consumer. This is questionable in the case of a dependent consumer. Also, many of the costs that might be thought of as private are actually redistributed throughout a household, a community and society through a variety of mechanisms and institutions. Thus, a case can be made that at least some of the private decision costs involved in the consumption of psychoactive substances are not offset by private benefits, and can therefore be included as part of the social costs of substance abuse. In sum, there is a theoretical difference between social and external costs, but in most economic analyses, external costs constitute all or virtually all of the social costs. In the case of substance abuse, most of the costs are generally also external costs, but there is some justification to include some private decision costs as well.

Why is so much attention paid to the distinction between private and social costs and benefits? As the Australian Productivity Commission report on gambling states (1999, p. 43), it is not because private costs are unimportant. In fact, often they are far more significant than the social benefits and costs of an activity. Rather, private costs generally do not justify government action on the basis that:

- individual actions based on adequately informed and rational decision-making will generally accord with the best interests of the individual concerned;
- if there are no impacts on other people resulting from these actions which are not accounted for, then what is in the individual's best interests will also be best for society; and
- if this is the case, there is no way that governments could intervene in individuals' decisions that would improve the welfare of either the individuals concerned or society more broadly (Australian Productivity Commission, 1999).

Thus the existence of private benefits and costs does not normally provide a justification for government intervention, unless the distribution of private benefits and costs is seen to be in conflict with society's concept of fairness. It can be argued that if lack of fairness is a problem it would be more efficient for the government intervention to take the form of broad social security or tax measures rather than measures targeted specifically at the activity under review. It may, however, be that a particular public sector intervention designed to reduce external costs will influence the size and distribution of private benefits and costs. In these circumstances public policy should not ignore private benefits and costs.

The key distinction appears to be between the private costs which rational and fully informed smokers incur by their own activities, and the social costs which are borne by others. However, the distinction is in reality more complex than this. Consider the case of a substance abuser, say a smoker. Conventional economic analysis of consumer behaviour assumes that rational consumers will undertake an activity only if the private benefits received at least equal the private costs of that activity, so that there is almost certainly a positive net benefit in the form of what is known as "consumer surplus" (the difference between what consumers would be willing to pay for a good or service and the market price that they are actually required to pay). Consumers are better off, in their own estimation, as a result of the consumption activity.

But this analysis refers quite specifically to the costs as perceived by the consumer. What if consumers (say smokers) are uninformed or misinformed as to the costs which the consumption imposes on them? For example, smokers may not be aware of the full health consequences of smoking (perhaps as a result of ignorance or of misinformation resulting from advertising) or they may not realise that the highly addictive nature of nicotine means that quitting will turn out to be much more difficult than they expected.

If the smokers' actions are determined by perceived costs that are less than their actual costs, the difference between the two is a social cost *even though it is borne by the smokers themselves.* This is because the smokers have not adjusted their behaviour in response to these unperceived costs and so these costs are unaccounted for. The smokers are not necessarily behaving irrationally. They are simply adjusting their behaviour to the best available, relevant information. It must be emphasised that costs borne by the substance abusers themselves can represent social costs *if these costs have not been knowingly incurred.*

It is sometimes suggested that these types of study should also estimate the extra value to the abusers (for example, the perceived benefits to smokers of smoking) over and above the costs to them of that activity, and that these net private benefits should be set off against the social costs. However, from the point of view of public policy, it is social costs that are relevant, not private costs. In determining the appropriate levels *for society* of any activity, government is interested in the costs that this activity imposes on the rest of the community. As an illustration, in determining the appropriate levels of activities such as pollution, environmental degradation or even violence, society does not take into account any private benefits that the perpetrators may enjoy. They are seen as being irrelevant to the interests of the community as a whole. In the same way, studies of the social costs of substance abuse should estimate only the net *social* costs.

In COI studies, only the social costs are considered. Some of the medical costs may fall upon the smoker if, e.g., there is a co-payment for public care or if smokers pay higher medical insurance premiums. Other institutional arrangements may require similar careful distinctions between the payments the smoker contributes to medical care (and other expenses) and the payments from other sources. These costs are not part of the costs-of-illness, but a part of the private costs borne by smokers, just as they pay the costs of their cigarettes.

Social costs may be incurred by other persons in the private sector (e.g., when private insurance premiums are increased due to payouts to smokers) as well as by public sector expenditure. Thus, in the context of COI studies, "social" is not a synonym for "public", nor "private" for "private sector".

Another issue which arises in relation to drug abuse, is whether costs imposed by abusers upon other members of their own family constitute private costs or social costs. On the one hand, it is argued (or asserted) that potential substance abusers will take into account the effects on other family members in deciding the extent of their substance abuse and that these costs are, therefore, internalised as private costs. On the other hand, how can we ignore the costs of substance abuse upon other people who have had no part in the initial decision and who may find the effects intolerable (for example, victims of family violence resulting from substance misuse) ? The size of abuse cost estimates will depend very significantly on whether family costs are treated as social costs. Practical questions will also arise about what constitutes a family member – de facto spouses, same sex partners, in-laws etc. It is, in fact, difficult to believe that the effects of substance abuse on other family members should be considered to be solely private costs.

Measuring the social costs of substance abuse is no easy matter. There is strong evidence, for example, that the consumption of alcohol is related to a variety of health consequences. The probability and severity of adverse health effects of alcohol are strongly related to level of intake, often in a non-linear fashion and sometimes in a manner which is also situation dependent (as with regard to accidents). The dose-response relationship is most evident with respect to cirrhosis of the liver, but adverse effects of high intake of alcohol have also been found for many other disorders including delirium tremens, impaired brain function, cancer of the oesophagus and digestive tract, chronic calcifying pancreatitis and congenital defects in the foetus among pregnant women. High and even moderate alcohol use is also associated with increased risk of trauma, such as that caused by impaired driving accidents.

The proportion of each of these causes of morbidity and mortality which can be attributed to alcohol use must be estimated, ideally for different age and gender groups. Where large-scale population based epidemiological studies have established the relative risk of particular disorders at different levels of alcohol consumption, the attributed fractions of alcohol-related morbidity and mortality can be determined with a fair degree of confidence. In many situations, however, such studies are lacking, and one is forced to estimate the attributable fractions from less reliable sources, such as studies of the excess morbidity and mortality among clinical populations. In such cases, one is forced to make the dubious assumption that rates of morbidity and mortality in the general population of heavy alcohol users can be estimated from clinical populations.

For other adverse consequences of alcohol use, the issue of causality can be even more daunting. For example, consider a person who consumed alcohol prior to committing a crime. Even if this person had been intoxicated, it is not clear whether the crime can be attributed to alcohol consumption. The alcohol may have caused the person to become aggressive or less inhibited, or precipitated the crime in some other fashion. On the other hand, the person may simply have happened to have a few drinks before engaging in a crime which he or she would have committed anyway. Alternatively, the person may have already decided to commit the crime and used the alcohol "for courage". Thus, even when drinking immediately precedes a criminal act, the attribution of alcohol as a causal factor in the crime is not at all clear.

Furthermore, the attributable fractions for each disorder vary between societies and within societies over time, so no one set of attributable fractions can be applied to all societies. Thus, the assignment of medical costs associated with adverse health consequences arising from the use of a particular substance such as alcohol is a very complicated and difficult task.

2.2.4 Further costs: productivity losses

The reduction in medical expenses in the counterfactual scenario is not the only important change as far as GDP is concerned. Total production may be increased because the former substance abusers are more productive at work, with lower morbidity and lower absenteeism. This additional production under the counterfactual scenario is the *productivity loss* from substance abuse in the actual situation.[6]

It is possible that to a certain extent, smokers may carry the burden of the lost production themselves, e.g. in lower remuneration. In practice, however, it seems unlikely that the entire burden of the productivity loss is carried by the smoker, and that at least some is carried by the employer in lower profits, by other employees in lower wages, and/or by the taxpayer in lower tax receipts. These losses are a part of the COI.

2.2.5 The ultimate cost: placing a value on life itself

There is one further major difference between the actual situation and that of the counterfactual which factors into economic cost studies. Substance use and abuse may cause death. Compared to the counterfactual scenario, the population is less. The resulting lower production should be included as part of the COI, by considering the loss of income due to premature mortality.

But what are we to do about the deaths of those who are not in the workforce, such as homemakers and the retired? It is insufficient to ignore this loss of life due to substance abuse. There must be an explicit recognition of the different life years experienced under the two scenarios. As discussed in Section 4, a dollar value can be assigned to the labour of persons outside of the workforce, and in the case of retired persons, some measure of the value of life years lost must be assigned. Better still life years should be adjusted for the quality of the living experience. Someone suffering from terminal cancer is not experiencing the same quality of life as their non-smoking equivalent who is leading a full life.

It is not easy to value these life years or *quality life years* (QALYs). Insofar as this is an appropriate thing to do, the difference between the actual situation and counterfactual scenario is a part of the COI.

The notion of placing a dollar value on human life is troublesome to many. Some cultures and religions could not contemplate doing so. What right have economists to place a dollar value on life?

Unfortunately, when it comes to policy advice, an economist cannot always avoid putting some value on life. Consider the question of whether to install traffic lights at a crossroad, one of which effect would be to reduce accidents which lead to deaths. If the evaluation ignored lives saved by the lights, that would be equivalent to treating the value of life as zero. As a result some life saving traffic systems would not be recommended. On the other hand if the value of life was set as infinity, every traffic system which reduced the probability of death, no matter how small that probability, would be installed, with the result that we could barely move given the density of life saving traffic lights.

So in practice we incorporate some value of lives saved, when we make policy decisions, even if a dollar value is not stated. All economists are doing explicitly is what others, policy advisers and policy makers do implicitly.

The issue of placing a value on human life cannot be avoided by ignoring the issue, for that would be equivalent to setting the value of life at zero. However, because economic cost studies do not strictly offer policy advice, they can avoid the issue by enumerating the number of years of life lost due to premature mortality without placing a dollar value on those years. For example, the result might be reported that the annual cost of a particular illness was US$ 100 million plus 10,000 quality life years lost. That meaning would be that under the counterfactual scenario, there would be US$ 100 million of extra resources for consumption, and 10,000 additional quality life years saved.

However the cost of another illness might be US$ 50 million plus 20,000 quality life years. Some may wonder which illness is the more costly, a question that can only be answered by combining the dollars with the quality life years in some way. Whatever way would be equivalent to putting a value on life.[7]

Another difficulty is that it is not clear that all life should be treated equally. This is especially pertinent in the context of substance abuse. Does the life of a chronically unemployed drunk driver have the same value as that of a young victim killed by the drunk driver? Does the life of a junkie have the same value as that of a productive, law-abiding citizen? The question of valuing the life of the junkie, compared to a good citizen, may turn out to be trivial, providing the counterfactual is kept mind. Suppose the counterfactual is to eliminate the substance abuse. Then the counterfactual scenario has the junkie as a good citizen, and her or his death is just as great a loss to society. Alternatively one might want to say the loss of the junkie's life is much less valuable than that of the good citizen, because the quality of life is lower. But, in addition, the counterfactual scenario is about the recovery of that low quality life to a standard one. Thus the total valuation, summing the two components, will be the same as the loss of the good citizen's life. The COI study includes the value of the existing damage to the life of an addict, as well as mortality effects.

2.3 Demographic approach vs. the human capital approach

There are two different approaches to the estimation of the economic costs of substance abuse: the more widely adopted "human capital" approach and the more recent "demographic" approach. The key difference, discussed in detail in Section 3, concerns the manner in which the costs of premature mortality are treated. In the human capital approach, the lost value of a deceased worker's production is estimated by present earnings plus a discounted rate of future earnings. The demographic approach compares the actual population size and structure to that of an "otherwise healthy" population, i.e. an alternative population in which there were no drug-related deaths.

The key point is that these different approaches are complementary rather than contradictory. The demographic approach addresses the question: "Suppose there had never been any substance abuse or problems associated with the use of psychoactive substances?" The human capital approach addresses the question: "Suppose all substance abuse and problems associated with the use of psychoactive substances were to end today?" The human capital approach generates an estimate of the present and future costs due to drug-related mortality in the current year, while the demographic approach estimates the present costs of drug-related mortality in past and present years.

Because these two alternative approaches to the estimation of the economic costs of substance abuse address different questions, it should not be expected that they would arrive at the same answers in all circumstances. During a period of increasing or decreasing consumption, one would expect somewhat different results. It is only during a prolonged period of stable consumption with no major impact from treatment or prevention programming that one would expect to achieve equivalent results.

Thus, there is no need to reconcile the two approaches. The need is to be clear about their origins and significance. The choice depends on the counterfactual situation being addressed. The preferred procedure will often be to conduct economic cost studies which utilize both the demographic and human capital approach, and compare the results.[8]

2.4 Prevalence vs. incidence based approaches

Estimates of the economic costs of substance abuse may be either prevalence-based or incidence-based. Prevalence-based studies estimate the number of cases of death and hospitalisations attributable to substance abuse in a given year and then estimate the costs that flow from those deaths or hospitalisations (as well as other costs, such as prevention, research and law enforcement costs). Incidence-based studies estimate the number of new cases of death or hospitalisation in a given year and apply a lifetime cost estimate to these new cases. Thus, prevalence-based estimates generally measure the costs of substance abuse in the present and the past in a given year, while incidence-based studies generally estimate the present and future costs of substance abuse in a given year. For ongoing health and social problems such as illicit drug use, the results of prevalence-based and incidence-based estimates are often similar. For health problems that are declining in magnitude (such as smoking in some countries), prevalence-based estimates will generally be higher than incidence-based estimates. For emerging health issues such as epidemics of HIV or Hepatitis infection, incidence-based estimates generally provide higher estimates than prevalence-based estimates, because many infected persons may still be in the latency phase of the diseases. The use of prevalence-based vs. incidence-based estimates is discussed in Section 3.11.

2.5 What economic cost studies are not

Part of the appeal and desire for economic cost estimates of alcohol, tobacco and other drugs may unfortunately be based on confusion with other types of economic analyses. While useful and relevant to policy decisions, COI studies are not studies of avoidable costs, they are not studies of budgetary impact nor are they cost-benefit analyses.

First, economic cost estimates do not indicate the amount of money and life years which could realistically be saved via effective government and social policy and programming. The counterfactual situation in economic cost studies is one in which there are no problems associated with the use of psychoactive substances. This counterfactual situation is hypothetical and generally not realizable under any circumstances. The estimated costs include both *avoidable* and *unavoidable costs*. Even if completely effective policies could be found with no appreciable costs for enforcement, treatment and prevention programming, implementation would not be instantaneous and there would still be lingering adverse consequences from past use of the psychoactive substances. The calculation of avoidable costs associated with the use of psychoactive substances is discussed in Section 3.

Second, economic cost studies are not studies of the budgetary impact of alcohol, tobacco and other drugs on governments. The costs included in COI studies are in reference to the whole of society and not just to the government accounts. A study of the economic costs of substance abuse would be very useful in conducting an accounting of the budgetary impact of psychoactive substances, as it would provide estimates for many of the government outlays. However, government costs do not include all of the costs imposed on the community. Further, budget impact includes consideration of government revenues and other benefits, which are not part of COI studies. The relationship between economic cost studies and estimates of budgetary impact is discussed further in Section 3.14.

Finally, economic cost studies do not attempt to fully consider the economic benefits of alcohol, tobacco and other drugs, and they should not be confused with cost-benefit or cost effectiveness analyses. These are two in a range of a range of tools that economists and others use to evaluate policy proposals. In the medical area they are frequently used to evaluate the usefulness of costly treatments or policy proposals (such as prohibiting drinking in certain circumstances) by, for example, weighing the costs of interventions against their benefits.

Cost-benefit analysis is based on the same value theory as COI studies, and economic cost studies can be used to provide important cost components in a cost-benefit analysis. However there are slightly different assumptions which means that cost-benefit analysis may give different outcomes and estimates. The most important differences involve the counterfactual scenario, and the treatment of the non-market sector.

Typically the cost-benefit analysis asks what would happen if the costs associated with a particular behaviour - such as tobacco smoking - were to cease from today. This contrasts with the counterfactual scenario in a COI study, which is to ask what would happen if the smoking had never started. Even if all smoking were to stop instantly there would still be the consequences of past smoking on mortality, morbidity, and health care. For instance the public sector would still be required to provide assistance for those who smoked in the past and were in need of medical care.[9] Such social costs are *unavoidable,* and so are not included as a cost in the typical cost-benefit analysis.[10]

The other major difference between cost-benefit analyses and economic cost studies utilizing the SNA framework is that cost-benefit analysis has been concerned with the impact of an event on non-market activities. For instance, if the a problem of substance abuse involves keeping patients in hospital beds, and a counterfactual scenario of returning them to the community, the cost-benefit analysis usually includes the extra unpaid work that might be involved in the second scenario (as when extra house and care work is imposed on family members).

The extension of economic cost studies to cover such unpaid and non-market activities does not represent a major difficulty in principle, but it has not been given priority in development. If economic cost studies were extended to include unpaid and non-market activities and if they were able to distinguish *avoidable* from *unavoidable costs,* it would be enormously helpful for those who wish to carry out cost-benefit analyses of alcohol and other drug policies and programmes. For an economic cost estimate is almost the benefit side of a cost-benefit analysis, and if done properly it could be readily adapted into the full benefit side.[11] The reason why the COI study is close to the benefit side of a cost-benefit analysis is that the avoidable costs associated with the use of psychoactive substances represent the benefits (i.e. negative cost) in a cost-benefit analysis contrasting the current situation with a counterfactual situation in which a policy or programme is introduced. Thus there are potentially strong practical advantages to integrating economic cost studies with cost-benefit analyses.

Thus economic cost studies, while based on the same value theory, involve differences with cost-benefit analysis. Some of those differences can be eliminated with development. There is no ultimate reason why the economic cost studies in the SNA framework should ignore non-market activities. Experience derived from cost-benefit analyses in dealing with non-market activities and estimating avoidable costs will hopefully inform the further development of economic cost estimates in the SNA framework.

Finally, it should also be noted that COI studies, like most forms of economic analyses, only concern economic costs to the legitimate market economy. There may therefore be significant economic costs in drug-producing countries arising from substance misuse that are not measured in the COI framework. For example, the costs of corruption are not generally included in COI studies. Nor do COI studies generally attempt to measure costs arising from the economic disruption to legitimate business enterprises caused by large-scale illicit drug production and distribution. To do so would require a more extensive and demanding economic framework such as general equilibrium modelling.

2.6 Interpretation of substance abuse cost estimates

Estimates of the aggregate costs of substance abuse tend to attract a great deal of political and public attention. However, while the meaning of individual components of the aggregate costs (for example, the costs of health care or crime) is relatively straightforward, the interpretation of the aggregate estimates requires great care and precision. To understand this point we need to return to the distinction between the human capital and demographic approaches to estimation.

Both approaches relate to the valuation of the loss of production arising from the abuse-related deaths of otherwise productive members of society. Both approaches compare production and abuse costs in the actual situation with those in a hypothetical alternative situation which would have existed had there been no past or present substance abuse. The difference between the two approaches relates to the way in which the production costs of premature mortality are treated.

The essential difference between the two approaches is summarized earlier in the following way. The human capital approach calculates the present and future production costs of abuse-induced deaths which occur in the present year. The demographic approach calculates the present production costs of abuse-induced deaths which have occurred in past and present years.

When looking at the human capital approach we are estimating the present value of the future time stream of lost productivity resulting from abuse-induced deaths. Although we talk of the "costs of abuse in year X", in reality a high proportion of these production costs will be borne in years subsequent to year X. In relation to the demographic approach, we are looking at the costs actually borne in year X but resulting from deaths not only in year X but also in many years prior to year X.

Thus, interpretation of aggregate estimates is difficult, but unfortunately there is no way round this problem. If we calculated the costs borne only

in year X as a result of deaths only in year X, the resulting costs would be very substantial underestimates of the overall costs borne by society since we would not account for the fact that deaths can impose costs over many years, not just in the years in which they occur.

One implication of the way in which abuse costs are estimated is that the aggregate figures are not likely to change significantly over short periods of time. This is because rates of abuse and disease prevalence, the primary determinants of abuse costs, tend to change slowly. Thus it may well be a waste of research resources to undertake these estimates at intervals of less than three to five years.

Some theoretical issues in the application of the framework

3.1 Definition and measurement of abuse

The definition of drug abuse is rarely attempted in the literature, and those definitions that are available are not usually expressed in economic terms. For example, the definition used by the Mayo Foundation for Education and Research defines abuse as "consumption of any drug for purposes other than that for what it was intended or in any manner or in quantities other than directed". It is certainly difficult to apply this definition of abuse to the consumption of tobacco.

A definition of abuse meaningful in epidemiological terms is that "drug abuse is deemed to occur when a relevant aetiologic fraction is greater than zero, i.e. when drug abuse adversely affects the health of the user". A more comprehensive economic definition, which encompasses non-medical costs such as accidents and policing, is that drug abuse exists when drug use involves a net social cost additional to the resource costs of the provision of that drug. Abuse occurs if the community incurs net costs as a result of drug use.

The measurement of abuse may require different measures for different drugs. The measurement of abuse is most straightforward for tobacco. While most tobacco consumption must be considered addictive, all tobacco consumption can be considered abusive since all tobacco consumption diminishes health status. Abusive drug consumption may be, but is not necessarily, addictive consumption. As an illustration, a road accident may be caused by abusive but not addictive consumption of alcohol. Harm minimization strategies for alcohol predominantly focus on the measurable effects of abuse such as health care costs and diminished health status, road accidents, and the costs of premature mortality.

These and related data can be quantified so that economists can cost the amount of abuse which can be attributed to substance use, but they do not provide definitive measures on the nature and measurement of abuse. For example, a recommended daily amount of alcohol consumption may be valid on a population-wide basis, but an individual may reach a level of abusive consumption well before or well after the recommended consumption level.

Indeed, an important issue in estimating the costs of alcohol is whether the counterfactual scenario is more appropriately no vs. low alcohol consumption. Different studies have adopted different strategies. The choice of low consumption vs. abstinence as the counterfactual can have a significant bearing on the relative risk of morbidity and mortality associated with higher levels of alcohol use. The use of abstinence as a reference category for relative risks is less complicated, but it may decrease the estimated relative risks of high alcohol consumption for those disorders with a "J" shaped curve (having lowest risk among low level consumers compared to abstainers and heavier drinkers). The use of low consumption as a reference category for relative risks results in higher estimated risks of high alcohol consumption for disorders with a "J" shaped curve, but it ignores significant risks associated with low level consumption for other disorders (e.g. traffic accidents).

When endeavouring to measure the abuse of illicit drugs, even less is known. Firstly, illicit drugs are not a homogenous category. In addition, the convenient definition that abusive consumption is equivalent to illegal consumption does not provide either an accurate basis for costing or a useful policy tool. However, while it may be much more useful to separate those costs which are incurred because of the legal status of a drug, e.g. law enforcement, not enough is known about abusive consumption of illicit drugs to produce a comprehensive measure of all other costs.

3.2 Definition of costs

The economist's definition of cost is based on the concept of an alternative use for scarce resources, known as opportunity cost. The measure of opportunity cost is the benefit which would be derived from the *best alternative use* of a particular resource. For example, the alternative use of land which is currently used for growing tobacco is the next most valuable crop which could be produced on that land.

A number of issues relate to costs, for which understanding of definitions is important. It is generally recognized that the costs of abuse include private costs and social costs, about which Markandya and Pearce (1989) say: "to the extent that the costs are knowingly and freely borne, they are referred to as private costs, but to the extent that they are not so borne but fall on the rest of society they are referred to as social costs".

In estimating the costs of drug abuse, other types of costs which require definition include tangibles and intangibles. Tangible costs can be defined as those costs which, when reduced, yield resources which are then available to the community for consumption or investment purposes. Intangible costs, which include pain and suffering, when reduced or eliminated do not yield resources available for other uses. As much of the efforts of the health care system are focused on the reduction of intangible costs, it is apparent that these costs are very important, albeit difficult to quantify.

It is also important to identify the concept of marginal cost, which is the increase in total cost attributable to drug abuse after allowing for the costs which would have otherwise been incurred in the absence of any drug abuse. In other words, this is a net cost concept.

For example, in costing health care, net costs include estimates of both incurred health care costs and potential savings. Those health care costs which are attributable to substance abuse should be set against the saving in health care costs which have resulted from the premature deaths of drug abusers. Had the abusers not died from causes related to drug abuse they would in many cases still be alive, suffering from other diseases and so imposing health care costs on the community. If abusers were not sick from abuse-related causes they would, in many cases, be sick from other causes.

It should also be noted that the resulting cost figures in COI studies are generally the aggregates of the individual costs which fall upon individuals directly or through agencies they have an interest in (such as the government). It is an assumption – a convention, rather than a scientific principle – that the sum of these individual costs are equal to the aggregate social cost. Any alternative convention is likely to involve more complex assumptions. The user of any social cost aggregate (indeed of just about any economic aggregate) needs to be aware of this assumption, and where necessary to go below it to a deeper level if the particular issue requires. The suggestion of disaggregating the total into institutional sectors (in Section 4) alerts the user to the aggregation issue and enables some insights.

3.3 Treatment and measurement of addictive consumption

Difficulties arise in practice in estimating the proportion of consumption which is addictive, although reasonable estimates can be made. There are strong grounds for the belief that drug use by addicts does not yield private benefits.

The theory of rational addiction, proposed by Becker and Murphy (1988), implies that persons contemplating the possibility of acquiring an addiction maximize their utility over time in the knowledge of the interdependence of present consumption and future preferences *and with full knowledge of the effects of the contemplated addiction.* In other words, the theory requires that potential addicts have full knowledge of all the drug's present and future effects at the time at which they are deciding whether to acquire the addiction. It is, considering the medical literature on the nature and sources of addiction, extremely difficult to believe that addicts make rational consumption decisions. It is even harder to believe that potential addicts have access to, and the ability to evaluate, all the relevant medical and epidemiological information in advance of becoming addicted, particularly when so many addicts are young or became addicted when they were young.

Ellemann-Jensen (1991) points out that total addiction has been assumed to imply that the smoker enjoys no utility at all from smoking but continues to smoke. He suggests that "such behaviour is clearly in contrast to the hypothesis of utility-maximization in standard economic theory". But, in fact, this is not necessarily the case. A 1991 editorial in the British Journal of Addiction suggests that addiction involves, *inter alia*:

- highly compulsive use;
- use despite harmful effects;
- relapse following abstinence; and
- recurrent drug cravings.

In this circumstance, the objective of drug consumption may well be to avoid highly unpleasant effects of withdrawal rather than to gain any positive benefits. Since the withdrawal effects result from previous consumption of the addictive drug, avoidance of these effects can hardly be viewed as a benefit of drug consumption. Short-run utility maximization need not necessarily imply long-term positive overall benefits from drug use.

The proportion of total consumption of an individual drug which is addictive consumption varies from drug to drug. For example, approximately 90% of Australian tobacco consumption has been estimated to be addictive but it is to be expected that the proportion of alcohol consumption which is addictive is considerably lower. The proportions applying to the various illicit drugs will also vary substantially.

3.4 Human capital and demographic approaches to estimating the costs of substance use

Two broad approaches have been adopted to the estimation of the costs of substance use – the widely adopted "human capital" approach and the more recent "demographic" approach. Both approaches relate to the valuation of the loss of production arising from the abuse-related deaths of otherwise productive members of society. Both approaches compare production and abuse costs in the actual situation with those in a hypothetical alternative situation which would have existed had there been no past or present substance abuse. The difference between the two approaches relates to the way in which the production costs of premature mortality are treated.

The human capital approach is to estimate the value of the worker's future production stream, brought back to present day values by the use of an appropriate discount rate. A thousand dollars received this year is worth more than a thousand dollars received next year (even if there is no inflation) because this year's resources become available for investment purposes a year earlier and so produce interest receipts or profits a year earlier. The use of a discount rate acknowledges this fact and adjusts for the difference between present and future values. Two major problems arise in the human capital approach – how to forecast future production levels and how to choose the appropriate discount rate.

The demographic approach compares the actual population size and structure with the size and structure of the hypothetical alternative no-abuse-population. From this comparison the actual and hypothetical outputs are compared to yield the production costs in *that year* of past and present substance abuse. The major problem in this approach is the estimation of the alternative population structure.

The essential difference between the two approaches can be summarized in the following way. The human capital approach calculates the *present and future* production costs of abuse-induced deaths that occur *in the present year.* The demographic approach calculates the present production costs of abuse-induced deaths that have occurred *in past and present years.* Which approach should be adopted depends, therefore, upon which type of information is needed. The two approaches are complementary rather than competitive.

3.5 Choice of appropriate discount rates

The estimation of economic costs associated with substance abuse applies to a particular period, typically a recent year. However, the effect of the counterfactual scenario may involve cost savings in later years. The standard economic procedure is to "discount" such costs in the future to an equivalent sum in the base period. The base period amount is smaller than the actual amount, even after adjusting for inflation, because events in the future are not given much (economic) value in the present.

The actual discounted amount can be very sensitive to the discount rate chosen. There is no internationally agreed upon discount rate, and even in a single country economists dispute the appropriate rate. These guidelines do not attempt to resolve this issue. Instead, it is proposed that where discount rates are required for the purpose of estimating the costs of substance abuse, the study should provide several estimates corresponding to different discount rates. While the preferred discount rate will vary between countries, it is further suggested that cost estimation studies include discount rates of 5 per cent and 10 per cent among those provided in order to facilitate comparability to studies in other countries.

3.6 Treatment of private costs and benefits

The overall costs to the community of substance use can be subdivided into private costs and social costs. If the costs of substance production and use are knowingly and freely borne by producer or consumer as the result of a rational decision-making process they should be classified as private costs. It can be assumed that, in these circumstances, there exist private benefits of production or consumption which at least equal the private costs.

There are three circumstances under which the consumer will not have rationally, knowingly and freely borne the full costs of the substance use:

- there may not be available full information as to the costs which substance use imposes on the user;
- the consumer may not make a *rational* decision based upon the costs of substance use which must be borne by the user;
- there may be no mechanism by which the costs which substance use imposes on the rest of the community (the external costs) can be converted into internal costs to be directly borne by the user. For example, it might not be possible for smokers to be forced to bear their full health costs or to provide recompense for the costs which they impose upon passive smokers.

Thus, if the costs of substance use are to be classified as private costs, the following three conditions must be simultaneously satisfied:

1. The users are fully informed as to the costs which the substance use imposes upon themselves;

2. The users are required to bear the full (internal and external) costs of the consumption; and

3. The users make rational consumption decisions in the light of all the information available to them.

These requirements are extremely stringent, so stringent in fact that the conventional approach of treating all abuse costs as social costs is fully justified.

3.7 Treatment and measurement of intangible costs, including willingness-to-pay methods

The major intangible costs of substance use to be considered here are caused by death, pain, suffering and bereavement. The most important characteristic of intangible costs is that, when they are reduced, there is no release of production or consumption resources for other uses. For example, any reduction of pain and suffering, while an important benefit, will permit no direct transfer of these benefits to any other person. An important implication of this characteristic is that there is no market in the benefits of cost reduction – the benefits cannot be bought and sold. Thus it is extremely difficult to place a value upon intangible costs and the temptation exists to ignore them. However, to do so may lead to misleading and unreasonable results.

To illustrate the potential problem involved in ignoring intangibles, take the case of the costs of smoking. A high proportion of smoking-induced deaths occur beyond the age of retirement, in which case the community receives a tangible benefit (forgone consumption exceeding forgone production). To ignore intangible costs could lead to the conclusion that smoking, by leading to the premature deaths of retirees, could benefit the community as a whole. The evidence that this conclusion is unreasonable is that most societies devote very considerable health resources to extending the lives, and reducing the pain and suffering, of people of beyond working age. They do not cease to be of value to society simply because they cease to work.

The valuation of life is quite generally attempted in many advanced countries – for example in benefit-cost analysis of road or rail investments. The two basic approaches to the valuation of life are the "human capital" and "willingness to pay" techniques.

The human capital approach estimates the discounted current value of the future stream of potential earnings of the victim. This approach undervalues life since it takes no account of the value of life to the victims over and above their earnings loss. To avoid death or sickness, most substance users would be willing to pay much more than simply their lost future earnings. The human capital approach can take account of this objection by arbitrary scaling-up of the estimated values but the theoretical basis for choice of the scaling factor is exceedingly weak. Nor does it simply include that many people make contributions to welfare even though they are not paid for it (as discussed later in Section 4.4.3). There can be a scaling up or imputation, but again the theoretical underpinning is weak.

The willingness to pay approach studies what people would be willing to pay for relatively small changes in the risk of death and from these figures produces estimates of the value of life. While this technique appears to have a much sounder theoretical basis, there still remain considerable difficulties in the accuracy and consistency of estimates using this approach.

Furthermore, when cost studies utilize a willingness to pay method for valuing life, it is no longer appropriate to compare the total costs of substance abuse to the Gross Domestic Product, as the total value of life using willingness to pay techniques is generally much higher than the GDP. One resolution to this problem is to compare the value of life in the cost of illness study to the total value of life in a society. This is elaborated in Appendix C.

3.8 Comparing and presenting estimates of the value of human life

There is no internationally agreed method of evaluating the value of human life. Some of the methodological differences include:

- some are based primarily on the loss of market productivity (which may be augmented by loss of non-market productivity);
- some impute a separate value of life above that of any loss of production, to reflect a human loss of death, pain and suffering. Common methods for doing so include measuring the number of deaths, or the decrease in the quality adjusted life years (QALYs) or the decrease disability adjusted life years (DALYs), valued by some monetary unit which may (or may not) be derived from willingness-to-pay studies. The use of QALYs and DALYs instead of deaths means that the assessment includes a valuation for deterioration in the quality of life while alive, while the number of years of life lost as a result of a death are given some weight. Thus, using QALYs and DALYs in preference to the number of deaths gives relatively higher social costs of abuse that is more likely to result in death at a relatively early age (e.g., from alcohol or illicit drug misuse) than where deaths occur at a later age (e.g., from tobacco use).

Different countries (and different economists) adopt different methods because, among other things their method:

- may be institutionalized by some official requirement;
- may be the conventional practice of the local profession;
- there may not be the data for the alternative method, or disagreement about key parameters;
- key data may be subject to an unsatisfactorily large margin of error.

This section is about where the value of human life includes an element in addition to that from the loss of production. It assumed that either the loss of material production (the tangible costs) has been treated separately in another calculation or separated out and that element is included in the material costs. However, for reasons described elsewhere it may still be appropriate to include an "intangible" component. The concern here is that if life is based on a willingness-to-pay method, for example, then the value of lost life numerically overwhelms the cost of material production. For instance, an estimate might find that the material costs (including loss of potential productivity) from substance abuse might amount to, say, 3 percent of GDP, but a value of life based on willingness to pay amount to ten times this figure.

The above point warrants further explanation. Gross Domestic Product (GDP) is the national accounting measure of production occurring in a whole economy during an accounting period (usually a year). It represents the value of goods and services produced in the domestic economy in that period. It does not include certain items routinely incorporated in estimates of the social costs of substance use. These include mainly intangibles such as the value of loss of life pain and suffering but also tangibles such as the value of unpaid work. To compare estimates of the social costs of drug abuse with GDP can be a misleading exercise since like is not being compared with like. Social cost estimates incorporating the value of loss of life can appear to be very high in relation to GDP because the value of life is not a part of GDP. It is an intangible, not a tangible and it is, in the economics jargon, a stock not a flow. It is, however, certainly possible to compare GDP with those components of the social cost estimates which are included in GDP estimates. This point is developed in Appendix C.

3.9 The positive economic impact of consumption

It is often argued (for example, by the tobacco industry) that if the industry producing the abused substance ceased to exist there would be a substantial social cost in terms of the resulting losses of output, income and employment. Thus the output, income and employment generated by the industry are represented as being benefits that the community receives from the production of the abused substance. However, this analysis rests upon two important assumptions, both of which are open to very serious question.

The first assumption is that, in the absence of any spending on the abused substances, the money would not have been used for any other form of expenditure – it would simply have been saved. This is highly unlikely. Most probably the money would have been spent on other forms of consumption that would have yielded very similar levels of output, employment and income.

The second assumption is that the resources used in drug production would have had no alternative uses. For example, the farmland used to grow tobacco would have been unsuitable for the cultivation of any other crop, and the farm labour employed in tobacco growing or in the manufacture of cigarettes would be qualified for no other type of employment at all. This assumption is also highly implausible.

The question does arise, however, as to whether employment would have been available for these people, in a situation in which there was substantial unemployment. If, however, as a result of the decline of the tobacco industry, only the *pattern of consumption* in the economy changes, rather than there being any decline in *total consumption,* any job losses in the industry will be broadly matched by job gains elsewhere in the economy. From a societal viewpoint, there is likely to be little change in levels of employment and unemployment.

An issue related to this is the question of whether abuse-related mortality causes any production loss during periods of significant unemployment since, it is often asserted, the dead can be replaced from the ranks of the unemployed who were not previously productive. Thus, the argument goes, in periods of high unemployment the production losses from abuse-related mortality are low or zero. Again it is necessary to examine the assumptions underlying this analysis.

It assumes that the skills of the dead workers can also be found in the ranks of the unemployed. However, one of the major characteristics of the unemployed is that they tend not have the skills demanded by employers. They are, in economic jargon, *structurally* unemployed. In many cases, therefore, the dead are not replaceable. The analysis also assumes that the unemployed are making no contribution to society in any unpaid capacity. Again, this is not a plausible assumption.

A difficulty with the assumption that abuse-related mortality causes no production loss in periods of high unemployment is that the calculated social costs of substance abuse fall as the unemployment rate rises. This means that the human capital approach necessitates the forecasting of future unemployment rates. This is a notoriously unreliable process since unemployment levels are partially determined by factors beyond the control of national governments, for example, changes in oil prices or in technology. In practice, cost estimates of abuse-related production losses are almost always made on the implicit or explicit assumption that the dead are irreplaceable.

3.10 Estimation of avoidable costs

It is assumed that the hypothetical alternative situation in which there is no drug abuse is simply that: hypothetical and not realizable under any circumstances. Estimates of the *total* costs of drug abuse comprise both avoidable and unavoidable costs. Unavoidable costs comprise the costs which are currently borne relating to drug abuse in the past, together with the costs incurred by the proportion of the population whose level of drug consumption will continue to involve costs. Avoidable costs are those costs which are amenable to public policy initiatives and behaviour changes.

An estimate of the percentages of mortality and morbidity that are avoidable was made in a comparative study by Armstrong in 1990. Armstrong (1990) uses an "Arcadian normal", which is the lowest age-standardized mortality rate for the relevant mortality or morbidity category amongst twenty selected, comparable Western countries. He implies that the Arcadian normal is the lowest percentage of preventable morbidity and mortality yet achieved in any of the chosen countries. This could suggest that no further improvement is possible. This appears to be an extremely conservative assumption, but nevertheless is a very useful tool for quantification of the percentage of preventable morbidity and mortality and their associated costs which can be reduced, and ultimately avoided.

Some of the identified costs of abuse, while avoidable, may be reduced or eliminated only over long lead times, which can be considered in three categories. Firstly, policy implementation lead times will not be effective instantaneously. Secondly, even after full and effective implementation of policies, there will be long lead times before the heath effects of policy changes are achieved. For example, the significant health gains from ceasing to smoke take between five and fifteen years to work their way fully through. Thirdly, as some costs apply to premature mortality, it will be years before the population structure reflects the avoidable reduction in abuse, and the associated avoidable costs.

3.11 Prevalence vs. incidence based estimates

A basic distinction between cost estimation studies is whether they are incidence-based or prevalence-based. In epidemiology, the term incidence generally refers to the number of new cases of a given disease or disorder that occurs in a given period of year (typically one calendar year) in the general population. An incidence-based cost estimation study uses an estimate of the number of new cases to estimate the economic costs in that one year and into future years. The essence of an incidence-based approach is the determination of a per-case lifetime cost estimate that can be applied to new cases. Incidence-based costs are quite important in performing cost benefit analysis (CBA) or cost effectiveness analysis (CEA). They portray and sum the magnitude of the economic impacts in each year of the individual's expected life from the date of onset of substance abuse. Thus, they provide us with critical insight into the value of preventing a case of substance abuse. This can be contrasted to the cost of preventing that case (whether through demand reduction or supply reduction). Incidence-based cost estimates may also be useful in the study of treatment, where the analysis begins at the age and date where treatment is initiated, and continues across their expected life. Incidence-based approaches have been used to estimate the costs of HIV infection and tobacco.

Many Cost-of-Illness studies, however, use a prevalence-based approach. In epidemiology, the term prevalence generally refers to the number of cases of a particular disease or disorder occurring in the general population at a given point in time. Rather than considering the life cycle of substance abuse as in an incidence-based approach, prevalence-based studies estimate the number of cases occurring at a given time to estimate the economic costs in a given year. Prevalence-based estimates therefore include for a given year not only the immediate costs of new substance abusers (newly incident), but also the costs of mature substance abusers and even of former substance abusers that still have problems (e.g., HIV, liver cirrhosis or respiratory illness) after they have stopped use of drugs, alcohol and tobacco, respectively.

Both incidence and prevalence-based approaches are useful for addressing somewhat different research questions. For example, in AIDS research both incidence-based and prevalence-based estimates have been used to address different policy issues. Incidence-based studies estimate the costs associated with new cases in the current year and into the future, while prevalence-based studies estimate the costs associated with past and current use in the current year. It should be noted, however, that those prevalence-based studies that use a human capital approach to estimate indirect productivity costs do consider some future costs in that these studies include estimates of the foregone productivity of those who die prematurely from substance abuse.

3.12 Crime and substance abuse

Certain types of crime involve no apparent "victim" and are sometimes termed "consensual" or "victimless" crimes. These are activities such as sex for pay, illegal gambling and the illegal drug trade. In some nations it is not uncommon to find some drug dependent persons in these professions. Consequently, in COI studies of substance abuse, consensual crime can make up part of the cost of crime. Economic resources used to enforce laws against drug possession and distribution are typically included in COI studies of the costs of illicit drugs. Similarly, some cost studies include an estimated cost for "criminal careers", based on the estimated value of foregone production by persons employed in illicit production or trade in abused substances.

In addition to these costs for consensual crime, the costs of some other crimes may be reasonably included in COI studies. There is little doubt that there is a strong statistical relationship between drug use and non-consensual crime. Criminal offenders have disproportionately high rates of illicit drug use. In Canada, for example, up to 80% of offenders report using illicit drugs during their lifetime, 50-75% show traces of drugs in their urine at the time of arrest, and close to 30% were under the influence of drugs when they committed the crime for which they were accused (Brochu, 1995). By the same token, drug users in treatment often have criminal records (see, e.g., Hall et al., 1993; Elnitsky & Abernathy, 1993). For example, more than four-fifths (81%) of Toronto injection drug users have been incarcerated since they began using intravenously (Millson et al., 1995).

However, the fact that a crime is committed by someone using illicit drugs doesn't necessary mean that the drug use caused the crime to be committed. There is clearly a relationship between illicit drug use and crime, but it is not always causal. There are several plausible causal connections between drugs and crime:

- The pharmacological effects of drugs: The consumption of certain illicit drugs might induce violent behaviour. Although many illicit drugs are negatively related to violence (e.g., cannabis and heroin tend to reduce aggressive behaviour), cocaine, other stimulants and PCP could produce violence by the loss of ego control, deterioration of judgment, induction of irritability and impulsiveness or the production of paranoid thoughts. However, the mechanisms for this relationship are in doubt and generally it appears that violence stemming from the pharmacological effects of illicit drugs is uncommon and cannot be attributed only to drug use (Abram and Teplin, 1990). Many, indeed most, drug dependent persons who commit violent crimes began doing so prior to becoming drug dependent (Kreuzer, 1993). This would indicate that the pharmacological effects of the drugs are at best only a partial explanation for their violent behaviour.

- The need for drug users to commit crime to support their drug use: Some people dependnet on heroin and cocaine are involved in crime to support their drug habits. For example, some sex trade workers may be involved in prostitution to support a drug habit and some dependent users commit property crime to support their drug use. These crimes are presumably committed because the addict's physical need for drugs is so strong that the demand for drugs is inelastic – no matter what the price, the user must obtain his or her drugs. However, the presumption that drug use invariably leads to crimes of acquisition is challenged by a number of observations. First, the majority of illicit drug users are not dependent. Second, most users, even dependent users, do not commit property crimes. Third, those dependent users who do commit property crimes tend to use drugs at very high levels, they have few legitimate sources of income and in the majority of cases they were engaging in criminal behaviour prior to drug use (Brochu, 1995). Third, the demand for illicit drugs is more responsive to price than is commonly believed: "An addict can use 2 grams on one day and nothing on the next. It is not the physical need that determines the amount of money needed, but the money available that determines the quantity of drugs consumed" (Grapendaal, 1992). Further, many former drug dependent persons continue to commit property crimes even when they no longer use drugs (Hammersley et al., 1989). As with the pharmacological explanation, this connection between drugs and crime undoubtedly plays a role in many cases, but it is only a partial explanation.[12]

- Crime results from systemic violence inherent in the illicit drug trade: There is little doubt that some crimes result from "turf wars" between rival distributors as well as arguments and robberies involving buyers and sellers on the illicit market (Roth, 1994). Systemic violence in the illicit drug market is most common in economically and socially disadvantaged areas that have traditionally high rates of violence. It should also be noted that drug dependent persons are not only more likely to commit crimes, they are also more likely to be victims of violent crimes and they have a high victim tolerance: "They do not renounce one another for fear, habit and self-protection" (Kreuzer, 1993: 78).

There is yet another connection that may account for most of the relationship between drug use and crime, but it is not a causal link. Many drug dependent persons adopt a way of life that accounts for both their drug use and their criminal behaviour. A number of longitudinal studies have shown that drug use and criminality are related to a similar set of socio-demographic and personality variables – e.g., poverty, poor future career or income prospects, and a low investment in social values (Brunelle and Brochu, 1995; Fagan et al., 1990; McBride and McCoy, 1981). There are undoubtedly many common underlying causes of both criminality and illicit drug use. Drug use and crime may well be mutually reinforcing, but according to this viewpoint, the real cause of both drug use and criminal behaviour are a complex set of underlying personality and social determinants.

There is thus little doubt that drugs are a contributing causal factor in some crimes, but the fact that a crime is committed by a drug user, even when he or she is under the influence of drugs, does not necessarily mean that the crime can be ascribed to drug use. The pharmacological effects of the drugs themselves account for few crimes, and a substantial proportion of crimes attributable to drugs stem from the fact that users must obtain their drugs from a violent and high priced illicit market. Much of the relationship between drug use and crime stems from the fact that some drug users have a lifestyle involving both drug use and criminality, and it is not at all certain that the criminality would not occur without the drug use. Like other "consequences" (e.g., violent crime, motor vehicle crashes, HIV infection) that may be partially attributed to substance abuse along with other factors, only some fraction of crime should be included in the costs. An attributable risk factor needs to be developed.

3.13 Who bears the social costs of substance abuse?

The 1994 First International Symposium on Estimating the Social and Economic Costs of Substance Abuse concluded that it would be desirable to indicate which community groups were bearing the social costs of substance abuse. A major reason for this recommendation was recognition of the fact that the incidence of these costs may change, even in situations in which the overall costs are stationary. For example, there is a significant international trend in the financing of health care to encourage a greater proportion of funding of health care by private individuals rather than by the state. Aggregate abuse cost estimates will not reveal this type of effect, whereas incidence estimates will.

Abuse costs can be treated as a form of tax and analyzed in a similar way. The costs can initially bear on one or more of four broad domestic community groups- the abusers themselves, other individuals, the business community and government- or they could be exported. As examples of these types of incidence of smoking costs we may cite the following:

Abusers – the physical and psychological pain of death from smoking-related cancers;

Other individuals – detrimental effects of environmental tobacco smoke (passive smoking) and some intangible costs (all intangible costs will, by their nature, be borne by individuals, either abusers or others; sometimes it may make sense to separate out the impacts on family and near relatives from the public at large);

Business – production losses resulting from smoking-related mortality, absenteeism and reduction in on-the-job productivity;

Government – funding of smoking-related health care.

Exported – drug-related increases in production costs could be shifted to foreigners in the form of higher prices for exported goods and services.

It is possible that these broad groups may be in a position to pass on the costs to some other group. For example, business may be able to pass on the costs of productivity losses to consumers in the form of higher product prices or to workers in the form of lower wages. This type of analysis is, however, fraught with problems since it is difficult (if not impossible) to know how costs are "shifted" in practice. Furthermore, all costs initially borne by business or government must eventually be borne by individuals (as consumers, workers, shareholders or taxpayers) either at home or abroad. Thus, incidence analysis should be confined to examining the initial burden of abuse costs among the community groups enumerated above.

It is important to appreciate that the social costs of substance abuse are not borne solely by the public purse. First, some costs may be incurred outside of the national economy. For example, there are substantial drug interdiction programmes funded by the U.S. government in South American and other Third World countries. While the costs for foreign programmes are included in U.S. cost estimates, it would be dubious to include costs paid by foreign governments in estimates of the costs of drugs for those countries in which the programming occurs. In a sense, these enforcement costs have been exported. More importantly, even when economic costs are borne domestically, a significant proportion of these costs may well be borne by individuals (for example, by the families or victims of drug addicts or by non-smokers exposed to environmental tobacco smoke). Again, in many circumstances, employers may bear these costs rather than government or the abusers themselves. Thus it should be appreciated that the following discussion on the budgetary impact of substance abuse relates to the impact of only probably a small proportion of total social costs.

3.14 The budgetary impact of substance use and drugs policies

In addition to the call which substance use places on real resources, it puts pressure on government budgets as a result of the need to fund such drug-attributable expenditures as health, welfare, drug prevention and the enforcement of drug laws.

However, the use of substances such as alcohol and tobacco also produces government revenue, mainly as a result of the high consumption and excise taxes that these products bear in many countries. Calculation of the impact of substance abuse on government budgets, therefore, involves estimating both expenditures and revenues resulting directly or indirectly from substance use.

On the outlay side of the drug budget there will clearly be increased expenditures attributable to substance use but there will also be some drug-attributable reductions. In particular, premature mortality resulting from drug use will lead to some reduction in welfare and health expenditures. Net health and welfare expenditures attributable to substance use will almost certainly be positive even after these "savings" are taken into account.

On the revenue side, in addition to the evident gains there will also be losses in revenue. Premature mortality will lead to reduced output, incomes and consumption and so to reductions in revenue from personal income tax, company income tax and indirect taxes. The major components of a study of the budgetary impact of smoking are presented below in Figure 1.

Extreme care should be taken in interpreting such estimates of budgetary impact. The results of these calculations certainly do not indicate whether drug users cover all the costs that they impose on the rest of the community. This is because some of these "external costs" do not show up as government expenditures (for example, the loss of production resulting from the health effects of passive smoking).

It could not be argued, for example, that "smokers pay their way" simply on the basis that tobacco-related tax revenues exceed tobacco-related public expenditures. Nor could it be argued that, even if the net impact of smoking on government budgets were shown to be positive (that is, smoking reduced the budget deficit or increased the budget surplus) then smoking was in the public interest. Budgetary estimates totally ignore, *inter alia,* the costs of loss of life, pain and suffering caused by drug use

A further type of calculation is the so-called "drug budget" which is a public policy indicator measuring the expenditure effort made by the state in the fight against drugs by adding the entire budgeted expenses attributable to drugs policies. Public decision makers in the drugs policy area almost universally have limited resources at their disposal. Measurement of government expenditures on the fight against drugs, the "drug budget", represents one of the main statistical indicators that can be made available to public policy makers. The drug budget should not be confused with the "social costs of drug use" which is an estimate indicating the resources which have become unavailable to the community because of drug use, and which could be used elsewhere if the drug problem was

FIGURE 1 – A DRUG ABUSE BUDGET

CHANGE IN OUTLAYS	CHANGE IN RECEIPTS
Increases	Increases
Welfare payments to abusers and their dependents	Sales taxes
Health	Value added taxes
Policing	Customs duties
Penal	Excises
Judicial	Other consumption taxes
Research	
Prevention	
Less decreases	Less decreases
Reduced welfare payments to abusers	Personal income tax
Health	Company income
	Indirect taxes (less subsidies)

suppressed. In the countries for which results are already available, the drug budget on average represents only about 5% of the social costs of drugs use. Nor should drug budget estimates be confused with the budgetary impact estimates presented in Figure 1. Drug budgets do not include social transfer payments. They only include direct government expenditures for policy costs such as treatment, enforcement, prevention and research.

Government expenditure on drugs can be classified into two types. On the one hand, there are expenditures detailed in public finance statistics, such expenditures as anti-smoking education and smoking-related research, which are directly related to drug problems. On the other hand, general authorities, such as the police, customs and public health institutions dedicate part of their resources to deal with problems generated by drugs, usually without specifically identifying the drug-attributable component of their expenditures. In almost all cases these authorities would not, in fact, have sufficient information to make such attribution. The evaluation of drug-attributable expenditures of this type is rarely attempted, yet they are undoubtedly an important component of overall government expenditures resulting from substance abuse.

In practice, such calculations are sometimes made in the field of the treatment of drug dependence. Administration of health costs reimbursement often results in the routine collection of cost data by diagnosis, which permits the development of cost estimates for health problems attributable to substance abuse. In contrast, the operation of policing and criminal justice often does not require separate accounting for activities resulting from substance misuse. Consequently, this type of information is not available unless countries finance special studies to estimate the attributable portion of such services resulting from substance abuse.

Not until the difficulties arising from the lack of statistical data have been overcome will it be possible to undertake international comparisons of drug budgets. For drug budgets to be compared, they should be expressed in terms of percentages of other standardized macro-economic aggregates. For example, the ratio of the drug budget to GDP or the ratio of the drug budget to overall public expenditure may be used as an indicator of the commitment by the state to dealing with substance abuse.

Comparison of overall drug budgets may also be complemented by an analysis of their composition. Drugs policy may be classified into two groups of expenditures: enforcement and treatment.[13] Enforcement expenditure relates to, *inter alia,* the costs of the running of the police forces and of the judicial and jail systems. Treatment expenditure relates to the sums dedicated to the treatment of the consequences of the drug consumption.

Examination of the balance of expenditures between enforcement and treatment by public authorities often shows that enforcement is the major component of the drug budget. This results not only from policy choices but also for statistical reasons. First, enforcement agencies (police, courts and corrections) are often more centralized than those giving medical care, thus making it easier to identify the expenditures for enforcement. In addition, court costs are often considerable and imprisonment is expensive, particularly when prison conditions are good by international standards.

3.15 Special considerations in drug-producing countries

The guidelines described in this report are based on the assumption that the factors of production used in local drug production (land, labour, capital, etc.) can easily shift into other industries if there is a reduction in demand (or, if the substances are imported, the foreign exchange saved is used for supplying other imports). The underlying methodology is what economists call "partial equilibrium". However in some cases the counterfactual scenario may involve a major adjustment to the economy (and society) because changes to the drug production sector of the local economy are sufficiently large to impact on the whole economy.

The assessment of the costs of substance abuse in countries with large-scale drug production would thus entails a more complex analysis using a "general equilibrium" approach, which is a well-established procedure for estimating the impact of –

among other things – industry closure. A general equilibrium analysis would provide an estimated value of GDP while the industry is functioning, and compare this to the estimated value of the GDP after the industry is closed down or reduced substantially in scale. The difference (after adjusting for price changes) is loss of social welfare, or the social cost of closure or scale reduction. While utilizing much the same principles as those on which the guidelines are based, this would entail an extension beyond the scope of these guidelines. Additionally, where the industry was operating illegally it is extremely difficult to quantify the effects of any drug-related corruption on human welfare, as well as institutional instability created by illicit drug production and other adverse effects (such as environmental damage caused by control measures). Because of such factors, the guidelines do not cover those cases where there is a substantial drug producing industry, although Appendix B elaborates some of the issues.

The geographical unit for evaluating the costs of substance abuse is typically a nation. However, the guidelines can be used to evaluate a smaller geographical entity, such as a province, state or region in a federation. It may be that illicit drug production in a smaller entity may have a significant impact on the local economy, in which case the remarks of the previous paragraph are relevant. Sometimes the geographical unit will be a group of nations. Again the guidelines should remain robust for that purpose.

Towards a common framework: the matrix of costs and issues of measurement

4.1 Which substances to study

Perhaps the first issue in designing a framework of what to include in estimating the economic costs of substance abuse is the issue of which psychoactive substances should be covered in the study. There is probably no right or wrong answer in making this determination.

Studies may reasonably focus on a single substance or on many substances. However, the determination of scope has definite implications in terms of the level of effort, the data requirements, and the analytic requirements. In practice, analysts have generally performed studies of the cost of abuse of and dependence on:

- alcoholic beverages;
- tobacco products;
- illicit drugs (other psychoactive substances) as a group; or
- alcohol and other psychoactive substances (but not tobacco), respectively; or
- alcohol, tobacco and other psychoactive substances, respectively.

Licit drugs such as prescribed medications and over-the-counter drugs, and volatile substances such as inhalants, are classes of psychoactive substances of epidemiological significance in many societies which have not been studied from an economic perspective. This would be a very valid and salient dimension of the substance abuse problem to analyze. Although the problems associated with misuse of licit drugs are not specifically addressed in these guidelines, they nevertheless present a valid and salient dimension of the substance abuse problem appropriate for analysis.

In situations where many persons use multiple psychoactive substances, it can be very difficult to develop estimates of the costs of particular substances. Good epidemiological and etiologic research should attempt to address this issue. However, the drugs and their patterns of use change continuously and rapidly, which makes it difficult to define and study consequences and costs associated with single substances.

In addition to determining which substances to consider, the scope of the study may be restricted to a particular drug (e.g., heroin, cocaine, marijuana), a particular mode of drug consumption (e.g., injection, smoking or oral), or for different potencies of substance (for any drugs under consideration). For example, public policy is often directed at the legal issues of a particular substance, such as decriminalization of or increased legal sanctions for a substance such as marijuana or powder cocaine or "crack" cocaine; taxation on smokable versus oral tobacco products; and differential regulation of beer, wine and distilled spirits. In theory this should be possible, although it may be difficult in practice because of data limitations.

The majority of economic cost studies have examined costs associated with the use and abuse of alcohol, tobacco and other drugs, respectively. Fewer studies have attempted to simultaneously analyze and compare the economic costs of multiple types of substances, or particular drugs, mode of administration or different potencies. Most studies of particular substances acknowledge the importance of examining and comparing the costs of other types of substances, but adopt a substance-specific focus because of limitations in time, resources or available data, or for the highly pragmatic reason that the funding source (often a government agency) has a substance-specific mandate. In sum, which substances and patterns of use are studied is generally driven by the needs of the sponsoring agency and the limitations of the data.

Each of the broad drug groups—tobacco, alcohol and illicit drugs—has particular problems associated with its cost estimation. Of these groups, the most straightforward for cost estimation is tobacco. Tobacco is invariably taxed in virtually all countries, resulting in reasonable records of sales and presumably consumption (often verified by household surveys). Morbidity and mortality data associated with smoking have been steadily accumulated and improving in quality and quantity. A number of countries have developed etiological fractions that provide an important tool for calculation and subsequent costing of tobacco-related illnesses and deaths. A further important factor in costing studies is that almost all tobacco consumption diminishes the health status of the user, and of others subjected to tobacco smoke and therefore does not require calculation of dangerous, neutral or beneficial levels of consumption. Tobacco studies are therefore generally able to be both rigorous and comprehensive.

The calculation of alcohol-related harm and concomitant costs is more complex, as some alcohol consumption causes harm, some is neutral and some is beneficial. Epidemiological work has provided the basis for calculation of benefits associated with alcohol consumption and for the health-related effects of harmful consumption. However, much alcohol consumption is neutral and involves no social costs. The non-medical component of alcohol-related harm (e.g., impaired driving, violence and alcohol-related crime) can be measured, but requires the estimation of attribution factors indicating the proportion of such harm that can be causally linked to alcohol consumption. Total alcohol consumption is more difficult to measure than tobacco consumption, due to various sources of unrecorded consumption such as illicit production, legal home production, and assisted production in "U-brew" and "Make-your-own-wine" stores.

The third group – illicit drugs – is the most complex to cost and the least likely to be rigorously and comprehensively analysed. Due to the fact that these drugs are by definition illegal, there are no taxes and thus no tax records. Illicit drug users are reluctant to identify themselves as such and barriers are created for treatment. For all these reasons, data on illicit drug use are uneven, incomplete, unreliable and sometimes non-existent. Crime attribution factors are difficult to obtain. In developed countries some crime costs are available, and usually some health costs, but these are subject to attribution factors. Researchers are usually reliant on survey-based prevalence data in the absence of official statistics.

Thus, recording systems provide a great deal more data on legal drugs such as alcohol and tobacco. However, in those countries where a significant proportion of alcohol and tobacco consumption stems from illicit importation or production, the estimation of alcohol and tobacco costs suffers from some of the same problems of data deficiency that apply to illicit drugs.

4.2 Major types of costs included in cost estimation studies

The use of psychoactive substances such as alcohol, tobacco and illicit drugs involves a numerous and varied set of adverse consequences. As indicated in Figure 2, there are four major types of costs that have been analyzed in economic cost estimates to date: (1) health care costs, (2) productivity costs, (3) costs to law enforcement and the criminal justice system, and (4) other costs such as property destruction from alcohol or drug attributable accidents or crime. Some of these costs have been omitted from certain studies out of data limitations--not from disagreements about the theoretical correctness of including such costs. Each of these types of costs is discussed in the following sections with regard to the potential for being estimated, and of thereby being included in a cost estimation study.

As indicated by the columns in Figure 2, costs may be tangible or intangible and the costs may be incurred by the individual user, other individuals, government or private industry. Intangible costs and the private costs to individual users are generally not included in cost estimation studies.

Most studies on the costs of substance abuse have found the three largest types of costs to be productivity costs, health care costs and those costs relating to law enforcement and the criminal justice system, which is why the cost framework uses these major categories of costs. This is but one of a number of different ways to categorize these cost items. Some of the cost categories in Figure 2 refer to efforts to "prevent" substance abuse, some are due to criminal justice efforts designed to "deter" or to punish problematic involvement with psychoactive substances, while others are the costs associated with negative consequences of using psychoactive substances. There are certainly other classification schemes for these costs, and the articulation of new or alternative formats could suggest other approaches to cost estimation.

It should also be remembered that the counterfactual situation in Figure 2 is one in which there are

FIGURE 2 – TYPES AND EXAMPLES OF COSTS ASSOCIATED WITH SUBSTANCE ABUSE

COSTS	PRIVATE COSTS (not generally included) COSTS TO USERS	SOCIAL COSTS (included in cost estimates)		
		COSTS TO USERS AND INDIVIDUALS	COSTS TO FEDERAL AND OTHER GOVERNEMENTS	COSTS TO BUSINESS AND OTHER PRIVATE
(A) Tangible costs				
1. Consequences to health and welfare system				
• Treatment for substance abuse	user paid insurance; out-of-pocket costs	excess insurance premiums	hospital + other health costs	contribution to health insurance
• Treatment for comorbidities and trauma	user paid insurance; out-of-pocket costs	excess insurance	hospital + other health costs	contribution to health insurance
• Prevention, research, health & welfare services			research, training, prevention, welfare	corporate research + prevention (EAP)
2. Productivity costs, i.e., consequences to the workplace				
• Premature mortality			foregone taxes	production losses due to premature death
• Lost employment or productivity	forgone income net of taxes	victims' forgone incomenet of taxes	foregone taxes	workman's comp., reduced productivity
3. Law enforcement and criminal justice costs				
• Criminal justice response	penalties (e.g. fines)	victim's time	enforcement, court incarceration costs	victim's time (productivity loss); criminal careers
4. Other costs, e.g., property destruction				
	unreimbursed property damage	fire losses, accident property damage	accident and fire prevention, fire	fire losses + accident damage to industry
(B) Intangible costs (not included in estimates)				
	pain and suffering to, user quality life years lost	suffering to dependents crime victims, + restrictions of public's legal rights to expedite		

no health or social problems associated with the use of alcohol, tobacco, licit or illicit drugs. The comparison of the actual situation to this counterfactual scenario does not consider certain opportunity costs which might be considered in different counterfactual situations. For example, if certain illicit drugs were made available via prescription or a government monopoly, there would undoubtedly be tax revenue for governments. Therefore some might consider lost tax revenue to be a "cost" of the current situation. However, the legal availability of these drugs is not the counterfactual situation in cost-of-illness studies, so forgone tax revenue is not considered a cost. In any case, tax revenue from drug sales simply represents a transfer of resources from drug purchasers to the rest of the community. It does not create any more resources for the community as a whole- it simply redistributes existing resources. Thus a loss of revenue cannot be a social cost, only a budgetary cost under a different counterfactual scenario.

As seen in Figure 3, there are a wide variety of health problems associated with the use of alcohol, tobacco and illicit drugs. Some of these are entirely attributable to substance use, while other causes are only partly attributable. The proportion of, say, liver cirrhosis deaths or traffic accident injuries, which can be reasonably be attributed to alcohol use will vary between societies and over time within the same society. Therefore the choice of the appropriate attributable fraction depends on reviewing the most current literature on each particular cause of morbidity and mortality. There is no one set of attributable fractions that can be applied in any society.

Regardless of how the various economic costs are classified, these are costs in the simplest economic

FIGURE 3 – SOCIAL COSTS ASSOCIATED WITH SUBSTANCE ABUSE WITH EXAMPLES

Costs	Costs associated with the use of		
	Alcohol	Tobacco	Other drugs
1. Consequences to health and welfare system			
• Treatment for substance abuse: hospital costs, physician fees, costs of medication + other health costs multiplied by appropriate attributable fraction	**100% attributable to alcohol use:** alcoholic psychosis, alcohol dependence, alcohol abuse, alcoholic polyneuropathy, alcoholic cardiomiopathy, alcoholic gastritis, alcoholic liver cirrhosis, ethanol toxicity, methanol toxicity, other alcohol poisonings **partly attributable to alcohol:** lip cancer, oral cancer, pharyngeal cancer, oesophageal cancer, colon cancer, rectal cancer, hepatic cancer, pancreatic cancer, laryngeal cancer, breast cancer, pellagra, hypertension, ischaemic heart disease, cardiac dyrshythmias, heart failure, stroke, oesophageal varices, gastro-oesophageal haem., cholelithiasis, acute pancreatitis, low birthweight, road injuries, fall injuries, fire injuries, drowning, aspiration, machine injuries, suicide, assault, child abuse	**100% attributed to tobacco:** tobacco abuse **partly attributed to tobacco:** respiratory TB, lip cancer, oral cancer, pharyngeal cancern, oesophageal cancer, gastric cancer, pancreatic cancer, larngeal cancer, lung cancer, bladder cancer, renal parenchymal cancer, renal pelvic cancer, respiratory carcinoma-in-situ, Parkinson's disease, ischaemic heart disease, pulmonarycirculatory disease, cardiac dysrhythmias, heart failure, stroke, atherosclerosis, peripheral vascular disease, phenumonia and influenza, chronic bronchitis, peptic ulcer, ulcerative colitis, low birthweight, sudden infant death syndrome, fire injuries	**100% attributed to drugs:** opioid dependence, opiate non-dependent abuse, opioid accidental poisoning, opioid cause suicide, other opioid poisonings, barbiturate dependence, barbiturate non-dependent abuse, barbiturate accidental poisoning, barbiturate suicide, other barbiturate poisonings, other drug dependence, other drug non-dependent abuse, other drug accidental poisoning, other drug suicide, other drug poisonings, drug psychosis, maternal drug dependence, newborn drug toxicity **partly attributed to drugs:** viral hepatitis, infective endocarditis, opiate caused low birthweight, HIV/AIDS
• Prevention, research and health services	Research, training, dependent welfare costs	Research, training, dependent welfare costs	Research, training, dependent welfare costs
2. Productivity costs: consequences to the workplace			
• Premature mortality • Lost employment or productivity	Production losses due to premature death. Workman's compensation, absenteeism, reduced productivity.	Production losses due to premature death. Workman's compensation, absenteeism, reduced productivity.	Production losses due to premature death. Workman's compensation, absenteeism, reduced productivity.
3. Law enforcement and criminal justice costs			
• Criminal justice response (including drug related crime)	Enforcement, court + incarceration costs; criminal career costs	Enforcement, court + incarceration costs; criminal career costs	Enforcement, court + incarceration costs; criminal career costs
4. Other costs, e.g., property destruction			
	Fire losses + accident damage, accident and fire prevention	Fire losses + accident damage, accident and fire prevention	

conception, recording the first instance of reallocation of resources in the economy. The key aspect of these costs is that either goods or services are used or delivered (direct costs) or human productivity is lost or impaired (indirect costs) due to an individual's use of psychoactive substances.[14]

Figure 3 does not distinguish between licit and illicit drugs. While desirable, it is very difficult to make this distinction because coding systems (the International Classification of Diseases, Version 9) do not distinguish problems due to licit or illicit drugs. For many categories, both licit and illicit drug problems are recorded in the same category.

The availability of data to estimate the following costs and concepts is often related to how clearly a particular type of consequence is related to substance abuse. In many cases particular services or problems are definitely recorded in administrative records as due to or related to substance abuse. Making estimates of such costs depends on gaining access to these data, and development of estimates will thereby be more direct and understandable to both the analyst and the ultimate user of the estimates. However, many adverse consequences arise from multiple causes in which substance abuse may or may not play a role. The analytic challenge is to obtain data that will provide a plausible basis for attributing some proportion of the costs associated with the particular negative consequence to substance abuse (the attribution factor).

The following discussion focuses on whether there are likely to be sufficient data to produce robust estimates of the major categories of costs associated with substance abuse. It does not attempt to detail all of the more specific costs within each major category of costs associated with substance abuse. The specific problems and their associated costs will vary according to substance – alcohol, tobacco and other drugs have different problems associated with their use.

Furthermore, the extent to which a particular consequence can be attributed to the use of, say, alcohol will vary according to setting, both for epidemiological reasons and due to variations in the institutional arrangements for dealing with adverse consequences. Thus, for example, the proportion of liver cirrhosis that can be attributed to alcohol will be strongly influenced by the rate of alcohol consumption in a society, patterns of drinking and the availability of treatment.

The establishment of the most appropriate attribution factors for alcohol and other drug related illnesses and social problems therefore requires detailed literature reviews for each consequence. See, for example, Holman and Armstrong's review of the appropriate aetiologic fractions for alcohol, tobacco and illicit drugs (Holman and Armstrong, 1990). Although such reviews do exist, the appropriate attribution factors conducted in one country may not be applicable to another country or even the same country at a different point in time. Therefore, the conduct of a cost estimation study on substance abuse requires careful line-by-line consideration of the specific costs to include and the attribution factors for each cost which are the most appropriate for the society in which they applied.

A further caveat regarding the following discussion of major cost categories is that it does not specifically address issues and methodologies for assigning values to indirect losses including premature mortality, morbidity and reduced productivity, crime victims' loss of work, incarceration and crime career losses. Studies tend to value losses of productivity using wage rates or replacement costs (for one's own business or for household productivity), with different values for individuals of different ages and genders. These issues are taken up in Section 4. The major objective of this section is to outline potential types of data sources and related analytic issues for each of the major types of costs in Figures 2 and 3.

4.3 Health care and health services

4.3.1 Treatment for substance abuse

This category of costs should generally have some of the most readily available data (although not necessarily comprehensive) about services delivered due to substance abuse. There are two reasons for this. First, some nations have identified publicly supported clinics that are dedicated to treatment of substance abusers. Therefore, there are government maintained data about the level of services and funding that are delivered through such service providers.

Alternatively, many health care systems collect data about the health problems for which patients sought and received treatment from hospitals, if not clinics, physicians and other health providers that do not specialize in treating substance abusers. These data are often recorded using an internationally recognized coding system (the International Classification of Disease, or ICD) that define alcohol- and drug-related diagnoses, including:

- dependence on alcohol or drugs;
- abuse of alcohol or drugs;
- psychosis due to alcohol or drug use; and
- poisoning or overdose from use of alcohol or drugs.

Thus a treatment episode or service received from a health provider can often be linked definitively to a substance abuse-related diagnosis and unambiguously attributed to substance abuse.

In the absence of system-level data that track the causes for which medical care is delivered (e.g., Holman and Armstrong, 1990), the analyst will have to find "special studies" that would provide credible estimates of these values. For example, particular hospitals or clinics might perform studies of what disorders were treated, and how much care they required. Judgment will have to be exercised in extrapolating such estimates to the entire system. For example, data from a "teaching" hospital that serves as a referral centre may not be typical of care delivered in many other hospitals, and it would be useful to be able to make adjustments to the data in order to address what may be known differences.

4.3.2 Treatment for co-morbidity and trauma

Excessive use of alcohol and drugs has been linked to numerous health problems, including, e.g., cirrhosis of the liver, nutritional and metabolic disorders, infection with HIV, motor vehicle and other types of trauma, and some mental disorders (see Figure 3). There are two challenges for the analyst in developing estimates of the costs attributable to substance abuse. First, it is necessary to estimate health expenditures related to these health problems. Then, it is necessary to develop estimates of the proportion of these costs that are plausibly attributable to substance abuse.

The ability to perform the first step depends on the development of data systems in a national health system. Again, where system-level studies have examined the level of services related to particular health problems using a comprehensive coding system (the ICD) it will be more possible to develop cost estimates for particular diagnoses (e.g., cirrhosis of the liver, or HIV infection). Without representative studies the analyst will need to make recourse to special studies (e.g., from a sample of health care providers) that must be used with caution.

The other major challenge in developing these estimates is to estimate the proportion of costs for a particular health problem that are attributable to substance abuse. It is rare that standard data systems would have the necessary data for this purpose. Studies in the United States of America find that medical records and data systems generally do not record whether or not a patient had an underlying substance abuse disorder that is likely to have caused the "presenting" health problem. Indeed, the analyst will need to identify special studies that have examined the underlying causes of particular problems, collecting detailed epidemiological information and undertaking analyses that attempt to identify the causal roles of various "risk factors".

The determination of attributable risk is particularly complicated for those disorders that relate to consumption in a curvilinear fashion. For example, coronary heart disease is lower among low-level drinkers than among abstainers. Due to this "J" shaped relationship between alcohol consumption and coronary heart disease, alcohol both causes and prevents morbidity and mortality. Economic cost estimates can subtract out the number of cases prevented, and thus present a net effect of alcohol on the number of hospitalizations or deaths due to coronary heart disease.
Alternatively, the analyst may choose to ignore the

number of cases prevented by low level consumption and present only the gross number of hospitalizations or deaths, on the grounds that a cost study should not give incomplete, partial consideration to benefits associated with alcohol consumption.

In estimating an "attributable risk" factor the analyst should carefully assess the rigor and depth of the research literature that is available on the role of substance abuse in a particular disorder. Studies of simple "association" (for example, the proportion of tuberculosis victims that were drug users) are not adequate for this purpose. They probably constitute the absolute upper limit of the role of substance abuse. Rigorous analysis will identify and adjust for the role of additional risk factors, and will almost always yield a lower "attribution factor" than the simple measure of association.

Also, better studies of attributable risk will use rigorous statistical standards in identifying whether or not risk factors (including substance abuse) are causally related to the health problem under study. It should be emphasized that there is no single analytic methodology that is most appropriate for undertaking causal analysis. There are a variety of "study designs" and methodologies that can produce useful information.

Attribution of mental illness to substance abuse is a perfect example of this challenge. Studies of drug and alcohol dependent individuals that are getting substance abuse treatment often find that up to a half of these individuals meet clinical criteria for various mental disorders ranging from depression, to schizophrenia. Likewise, studies of the mentally ill find that material proportions have substance abuse problems.

However, there is uncertainty about the causal relationship of the two types of disorders. Some research shows that mentally ill individuals initiate or escalate drinking and drug taking presumably to "self medicate" their disorder. Yet other research finds that alcohol and drug abusers develop symptoms of certain mental disorders (e.g., depression, anxiety, psychosis) as their substance disorder becomes more severe, when they abuse particular substances (alone or in combination) or when they attempt to stop using or detoxify. The challenge in developing attributable risk" factors for mental disorders (and for the costs of treating mental disorders) is to estimate how much of the treatment for mental disorders is caused by substance abuse—not simply associated with substance abuse. If an already severely mentally ill individual develops a substance abuse disorder, the additional care that such an individual requires should be attributable to substance abuse, however the expected care for the mental disorder apart from the substance abuse problem would not be attributable.

4.4 Productivity costs

In most COI studies estimating the costs of substance abuse, the largest cost involves lost productivity due to premature death, disability, absenteeism and other causes of lower productivity on the job. Estimation of productivity costs requires, first and foremost, robust estimates of premature mortality and morbidity that can be attributed to substance abuse.

4.4.1 Premature mortality

National health systems view data about mortality as quite valuable in monitoring the health of the populace. Often mortality data (deaths for one or more year) are centrally collected, with information about the cause of death and demographic characteristics of the decedent. Cause of death can be coded for purposes of analysis using the ICD system. As noted above, there are identified ICD substance abuse-related codes that can be associated with deaths. When national mortality data are collected and processed in this form it makes the task of the analyst relatively straightforward in assembling data on deaths with a direct link to substance abuse.

However, substance abuse can also cause death indirectly, as discussed above under "Health Treatment for Comorbidities and Trauma". As indicated previously, the challenge to the analyst is to first identify causes of death for which there is research substantiating a causal role for substance abuse, to obtain the data on mortality for the year(s) of concern related to that cause, and then to develop and estimate of the proportion of deaths that are attributed to substance abuse. The same analytic issues apply to studies of mortality as to studies of health care utilization. Greater reliance should be put on more "rigorous" studies. Studies of "association" should be eschewed in favor of studies analyzing the contribution of multiple risk factors that apply standard statistical criteria to the analysis.

4.4.2 Morbidity – lost employment or productivity

There are real economic losses associated with illness-caused lost days of work (in paid employment, in one's own business such as agriculture, and in household productivity), and with work performed (in any of these venues) by those that have long-term or short-term impairments or disabilities. Measuring and attaching values to these phenomena is quite challenging for many of the same issues that must be addressed in estimating health care resources used to address substance abuse. This discussion does not address issues primarily related to valuation of lost or impaired work time, such as what is the unemployment rate in the nation under study. These estimates should be understood to represent lost or reduced "potential" work time/productivity.

The first type of data concerns work time missed due to participation in treatment. Residential, hospital and "day treatment" patients usually miss work, and to the extent that data exist on care delivered in such settings it is possible to develop basic estimates of lost work time. Similarly, participation in ambulatory or outpatient treatment may entail some time away from work to receive treatment, and this estimate can be constructed with data on enrollment in outpatient treatment. These data should also include information about the demographic characteristics of the patients, in order to make adjustments for the "expected" level of employment/productivity.

Another source of data would come from estimates of patient time spent in hospital and ambulatory health care for health problems caused by substance abuse. This would build on the same analytic literature and data used to make estimates for health care services above.

A further source of data for this estimate would be from studies of health and employment. For example, health surveys in the United States of America ask about health status, loss of work due to health problems, and the nature of those problems. Health problems are coded for analysis using the ICD system, and data can be assembled on diagnoses that are directly coded as substance abuse, and for health problems/diagnoses that have been established as related to/caused by substance abuse in the epidemiological and etiologic literature.

Prior studies have found that the largest part of morbidity/lost and reduced productivity costs is not due to measurable lost days of work, but from impaired productivity while on the job. Numerous studies have found that many substance abusers hold jobs. There is a smaller, but growing literature that has yielded evidence that substance abusers are less productive in their jobs than individuals with otherwise similar experience and capabilities.

Such studies use labour economics models to analyze "general population" surveys that contain standard labour market information as well as information about use of and problems associated with psychoactive substances. The objective of such an analysis is to use statistical analysis to identify patterns of substance use or problems that are associated with employment and earnings deficits, standardizing or controlling for the other characteristics of substance abusers. These estimates are then applied to estimates of the proportion of the population (employed and otherwise) that have these patterns of use or problems, and then to assign economic values to the identified deficits.

It is widely recognized that substance abuse by workers can adversely affect their performance and the productivity of the workplace. However, there is a major theoretical and empirical problem when one attempts to estimate the cost of substance abuse on the workplace. The effect of employers operating in markets for labour, other inputs, capital and wages for goods and services serves to spread the impacts between the employers (lost profits), the workers (lost earnings and benefits) and consumers (higher prices for goods and services). The distribution of costs between these parties can not be determined solely by using economic theory, since the outcome is partly determined by market conditions and, in particular, by the relative bargaining abilities of employers, workers, and consumers.

In theory, the value of workers to the employer is determined by calculating the amount that they work times the value of their productivity when they work. In a perfectly functioning labour market, workers' wages are expected to equal the value of their productivity to the enterprise. Earnings are by definition the amount of time worked times the wages paid per amount of time.

Substance abuse by workers can affect both the amount of time that they work (e.g., missed time due to absenteeism, tardiness, excess sickness) and their productivity when they are at work (e.g., lower quality of their efforts, costs of mistakes caused by substance misuse). It is also emphasized that worker problems can adversely impact the productivity of co-workers and managers, as well as morale in the workplace when other employees must work harder or otherwise deal with problems caused by substance misuse.

If the labour market were working perfectly, any reduction in productivity resulting from the worker's substance abuse would result in a reduction in the wages that the employer was willing to pay that worker. This type of analysis has lead some economists to conclude that the costs of substance abuse by workers are borne by the workers themselves in the form of lower wages. Thus, this line of reasoning concludes, these costs are private costs borne by the workers, not social costs borne by the rest of the community.

This analysis also implicitly assumes that the workers have made rational and fully informed decisions to become substance abusers, in most cases a dubious assumption. An even more serious problem affecting the above conclusion is the underlying assumption that labour markets function perfectly so that virtually automatic wage or salary adjustments occur as a result of productivity declines caused by substance abuse. In practice, the validity of this assumption depends very much upon the institutional and other characteristics of the country for which the cost estimates are being made. Labour markets may not work perfectly for a variety of reasons:

- Employers may not recognise the abuse-associated costs which they are bearing.
- Wages may not be flexible downwards for institutional reasons. For example, Australia has a system of award rates and conditions which drastically reduces the scope of downward flexibility.
- Unfair dismissal legislation may make it difficult to dismiss less productive workers.
- The abusers may be employed in the public sector where wage flexibility may be much lower and dismissal procedures much more cumbersome.
- The abusers may be employed by companies which have organisational slack (that is, have not minimised costs for their chosen output levels) and which have the ability to pass on higher costs to their customers in the form of higher prices. Markets may not be sufficiently competitive to ensure that firms with organisational slack will ultimately fail.

To summarise, only where labour markets are functioning perfectly will substance abuse-attributable production costs be totally private costs (assuming that the other necessary conditions are also met). Analysis of the incidence of workplace costs (that is, in which sector(s) those costs are borne) requires that serious attention should be paid to the institutional characteristics of the relevant labour market.

This type of costs applies primarily to "health-related" impacts on employment. As will be discussed later, substance abuse has other avenues through which it appears to impact on labour market performance and productivity – mainly related to criminal activities and incarceration of criminals.

4.4.3 Treatment of non-workforce mortality and morbidity

The valuation of production lost as a result of substance use could be taken to be the value of wages forgone, on the basis that wages are equal to the worker's productivity (this value is often taken to be average earnings) or on the basis of some estimate of average gross domestic product per worker. However, this approach to costing is unsatisfactory because it does not assign any value to the unemployed, the retired or women outside the paid workforce, since they do not earn wages or salaries. People not in paid employment may well be contributing output but it is unpaid work, and so its value is not incorporated in conventional measures of national output

This issue can be clarified by use of the distinction between tangible and intangible costs. There will be no loss of *paid* output as a result of morbidity or mortality of the unemployed, the retired, children, students, parents at home looking after children, or other people not in the workforce but there will be a value of lost *unpaid work,* as well as the loss of life incurred by these people themselves. There will also be a loss of unpaid work as a result of deaths of the employed but, according to available evidence, this loss will on average be less than for the rest of the adult population. The deaths of both employed and unemployed/out-of-the-work-force will impose a social cost but the cost will be greater for the employed. This point is illustrated in Figure 4.

In summary, for the employed the net cost is the loss of paid output *plus* the loss of unpaid output *plus* the value of life. For the unemployed or people out of the work force, the net cost is the loss of unpaid output *plus* the value of life. This analysis clearly disposes of the suggestion that society incurs no cost as a result of the premature deaths of the unemployed or people out of the work force.

Estimates of the value of unpaid work place a value on these activities that could have been replaced by an equivalent service purchased from an outside source. For, example, the child-minding activities of "non-working" mothers might be replaced by hired nannies. The types of activities to be considered here are domestic activities, childcare, purchasing of goods and services, and volunteer and community work. The sickness or death of people engaged in such activities will involve withdrawal of others from the workforce to maintain the supply of non-market services. Value can be placed on these activities by estimating the cost of hiring a market replacement for each individual function. In this way the important issue of the value of productivity of married women in the family home is satisfactorily handled.

The use of average earnings to indicate the value of the lost output of the employed implies that it represents the value of the output of the sick or prematurely dead. In practice, average earnings may be below the value of output because of labour market imperfections or because the workers involved are not paid the full value of their output. In addition, weekly earnings as measured by national statisticians tend to omit some important components of earnings, for example superannuation and fringe benefits, and the incomes of proprietors and partners of unincorporated busi-

FIGURE 4: THEORETICAL IMPACT OF PREMATURE MORTALITY

Death of	Tangible cost	Tangible benefit	Intangible cost	Intangible benefit
Employed	• Loss of paid output • Loss of unpaid output	• Reduction of consumption	• Reduction of consumption • value of life	nil
Unemployed or out of work	• Loss of unpaid output	• Reduction of consumption	• Reduction of consumption • value of life	nil

ness and of self-employed people. Adjustments should, therefore, be made for those other components of income.

4.5 Crime and law enforcement costs

4.5.1 Criminal justice expenditures

As for health care expenditures, some criminal justice services are identifiably and by definition related to use of psychoactive substances, while others are indirectly, although still causally related to use of psychoactive substances. One may think of three different types of cost estimation situations with respect to the various types of criminal justice services: criminal justice activities completely dedicated to combat the consequences of use of psychoactive substances (such as a distinct alcohol or drug enforcement unit); activities by general criminal justice entities that address illegal use of psychoactive substances; and activities of general criminal justice entities to address crimes believed to be caused by use of psychoactive substances. Estimates can theoretically be developed for law enforcement authorities (police and prosecutors), courts, and corrections (prisons, jails, and community supervision of offenders).

Data on criminal justice units that are solely or predominantly dedicated to address illegal use of psychoactive substances can usually be obtained from government sources. These are the least ambiguous of the criminal justice costs, if such units exist and data are available.

The greater challenge comes in analyzing costs from general criminal justice entities, particularly law enforcement and judicial services. It is very difficult to allocate effort and costs across the different missions of such entities. For law enforcement there may be data about types and numbers of arrests, for example about infractions against alcoholic beverage laws, or drug control laws, respectively. These arrest data provide a first level to allocate effort and costs across various types of offences. However, this raises the question of how much effort and cost is involved with an arrest for each type of offence. Such data are likely to be unavailable, and it will probably be necessary to make and acknowledge simplifying assumptions about cost allocations.

The most difficult cost estimates will involve making attributions of the role of using psychoactive substances in other types of crime such as robbery, burglary, assault, prostitution and gambling. Mankind has spent eons contemplating why we break social norms (commit crimes), much attention is being given to the use of psychoactive substances. It should be sufficient to say that data about the proportion of offenders that were intoxicated with alcohol or drugs when they committed a crime are only data about association, and provides circumspect information about causation.

The analyst must be very careful and explicit in discussing how attribution factors are derived for such crimes. It may often come down to whether the analyst is willing to exercise their reasoned judgment and make an explicit assumption about the rate. If so, that assumption should be backed up by a chain of logic and the best data that are available.

4.5.2 Crime victim's time losses

A material, if relatively small, share of costs is derived from lost work experienced by crime victims. Estimates of this type of cost depend on having data about the number of crimes experienced by victims per year, data about the amount of productive work time lost due to a crime (at a job, one's own business, or in the household), and the proportion of various types of crimes that are attributed to use of psychoactive substances.

Basic data about the number of crimes might be accumulated and reported by criminal justice authorities but it should be understood that these data are probably a dramatic underestimate of the amount of crime. Studies have shown that the largest proportion of crimes (e.g., assaults and theft) are never reported to criminal justice authorities by the victims. Studies of crime victims should be used to develop estimates of how many crimes are experienced and what level of work disruption is experienced. Such data usually come from the same studies that examine property loss and destruction associated with crime (see above).

This still requires the analyst to confront the issue of attribution of crimes to use of psychoactive substances.

4.5.3 Incarceration

When individuals are incarcerated they are often partially or totally removed from the productive economy. This constitutes a loss of potential productivity to the economy. While this loss represents a conscious decision by society, deemed to be justified on the basis of protecting other citizens and punishing offenders, it is nonetheless a withdrawal of a certain number of the populace from the possibility of participating in productive activities. This withdrawal, or loss, is reduced to the extent that prisoners engage in work while incarcerated, either for outside purposes, or to support the prison.

Data about incarcerated populations (and the costs of operating those systems) should be more readily available and more reliable than data about law enforcement activities. Information should be collected about those that are incarcerated due to crimes defined as due to use of psychoactive substances (violations of alcohol beverage control laws, and use and trading in controlled substances) and crimes where there is some attribution role for psychoactive substances. In the latter case data on incarcerated persons should be obtained by type of offence, as the extent of involvement (and attribution) of psychoactive substances is likely to vary.

One type of study that an analyst should seek in developing this estimate is a survey of prison inmates. Sometimes such studies undertake to analyze factors believed to be involved with criminal behaviours, included whether the individual has a history of use of psychoactive substances, or was using them at the time that they committed the crime for which they are incarcerated. As before, the analyst should attempt to arrive at estimates judged to reflect "causality" relying if possible on data and analysis, but always it will be necessary to use careful judgment.

4.5.4 Crime career costs

This is probably the most esoteric and ephemeral of the costs associated with use of psychoactive substances, and probably the most difficult to estimate. The concept behind "crime career" costs is that some otherwise able-bodied and able-minded users of these substances "drop out" of the legal economy in order to produce or trade in psychoactive substances or to pursue income-generating crime because of the demands of their drug addiction. Thus there is a loss of potential production in the legitimate economy.

It is extremely challenging to estimate this cost component, and it would be an understatement to say that the estimates would have poor statistical reliability. This estimate would probably have little or no statistical properties because the estimates used for this cost may have to be based on expert judgments and informed opinions. There have been few studies that have produced statistically rigorous and plausible estimates of the size of this population.

Data of some nature may exist for various parts of this population, such as addicts seeking treatment or health care, or drug users and traffickers that are arrested. Such data can be combined to generate lower-bound estimates of the size of the population under discussion, however, anthropological studies of this population find that a surprisingly large proportion of addicts have never been in treatment, sought health care, or arrested. Also, studies have attempted to use sophisticated statistical inferential techniques to indirectly estimate the size of the population (for example, the capture-recapture model, and epidemiological models of transmission of HIV infection among injection drug users).

The analyst may need to search extensively in order to develop such estimates. Ultimately it will become a question of judgment about which data to use, if any, and how to combine estimates from disparate sources. The most meaningful test for this estimate, if it is developed, is whether it is judged to be credible – not statistically rigorous – by those who have carefully studied the problem from various perspectives.

4.6 Other costs

4.6.1 Treatment of research, education and law enforcement costs

Some costs that are clearly attributable to substance use result from public decisions to reduce abuse rather than being the direct effects of substance use. Costs in this category include expenditures on research on the impact of substance use, public education campaigns to minimize use or abuse, and law enforcement programs to reduce illegal dealing and use. These costs are discretionary in the sense that governments could choose not to incur them, or, indeed, to incur higher levels. It is to be expected that reduced expenditures would lead to higher direct costs of substance use but these expenditures are, nevertheless, not themselves direct costs.

It is appropriate to indicate the level of social costs incurred in these expenditure areas but to categorize them as "policy costs" rather than direct costs. They are, in this way, identified as being incurred in relation to substance use but are not classified as unavoidable costs of use.

4.6.2 Prevention and other public health efforts

The primary source of data on this item will generally be from government budgets. Many of these services are in the form of media messages, educational efforts and materials. However, other services and activities are also considered to be useful in combating substance abuse, such as after school activities for adolescents, and interventions with youth at risk of school drop out of failure. Consequently, funding of these services may be motivated by the substance abuse problem and therefore recorded as part of the effort to address substance abuse. However, the 1994 First International Symposium on Estimating the Social and Economic Costs of Substance Abuse recommended that these costs should be recorded as discretionary policy costs rather than as unavoidable costs of substance abuse, because the counterfactual is likely to have them continue, after the abuse is reduced or even ceased.

4.6.3 Property destruction or losses due to crime or accidents

The inclusion of the cost of property destroyed or the reduction in value due to accidents caused by substance abuse is relatively uncontroversial. Property losses due to crime caused by substance abuse is somewhat more contentious. While the transfer of ownership via a theft is usually treated as an economic transfer and therefore not a cost to the economy as a whole, the stolen property typically has significant lower value than it had before it was stolen. In such cases, the cost evaluation procedure should follow the local practice, i.e., take into account the fact that theft results in a reduction in value of property. This should be explicitly mentioned and the reduction in value of stolen property itemized in the cost calculations.

There are two sets of data necessary to estimate the costs of property damage due to crime or accidents caused by substance abuse. The first is data on the incidence and costs of such events, and the second is a set of estimates about the proportion of the national total that can be attributed to substance abuse (whichever substances are under examination).

National data on total incidence and costs for these impacts will generally come from, respectively, criminal justice system studies on the incidence and nature of crime, and from a system that tracks events such as motor vehicle crashes and fires. Both property and personal crime sometimes involve damage to and destruction of property, although this value seems to be relatively small, compared to other costs associated with substance abuse. On the other hand, property damage from motor vehicle crashes, fires, other transportation accidents (train, air) can amount to sums orders of magnitude greater than that involved with crimes. These data may be either maintained in a regularly operating reporting system (probably sponsored by a government agency), or collected through special studies performed on an irregular basis.

To complete these estimates there must be research on the involvement if not the causal role of substance abuse in the respective causes of property damage. While reporting systems on motor vehicle (and other transportation) crashes do increasingly assemble and report data about the involvement of alcohol and other psychoactive substances, this is less likely to be true for other causes of property damage. Accordingly, recourse will need to be made to the epidemiological literature for special studies of these problems with the general caveats for utilization of such studies.

Note that it would generally not be appropriate to use attribution factors for one cause of damage to another. Different types of crime typically involve alcohol and other psychoactive substances to varying degrees, and the same has been found in motor vehicle crashes of different severity. Fatal motor vehicle crashes have generally been found to be much more likely to involve operator consumption of alcohol than are non-fatal crashes.

4.6.4 Welfare costs

In dealing with the welfare costs attributable to drug abuse great care needs to be taken to distinguish between the real resource costs of abuse and costs which are simply pecuniary costs (i.e. transfer payments). The welfare costs dealt with here relate to the payments borne by the state (such as invalid pensions and sickness benefits). Relevant welfare payments are made to the victims of drug abuse, their carers and dependents.

Welfare cost calculations should also incorporate some estimate of the proportion of the total administrative costs of the social welfare system that is attributable to substance abuse-related welfare dependence. These administrative costs are real resource costs and should always be counted.

It is important to ensure that there is no double counting of costs or benefits. If a person previously in the workforce receives welfare benefits as a result of abuse-related sickness it would be double counting to include in the estimate of social costs both the productivity loss and the direct cost of welfare benefits. The productivity loss is a real resource loss while the welfare payment simply represents a redistribution of consumption ability from the rest of the community to the abuser. However, if the abuser is rational and fully informed the private resource costs will be fully internalised and should not be counted as part of social costs. On the other hand, in these circumstances the welfare costs will represent an externality imposed on the rest of the community and should be incorporated in social costs. It is never correct to count both productivity and welfare costs. Which should be counted depends on the assumptions about the rationality of, and the amount of information available to, the abuser. All welfare costs should be incorporated in estimates of budgetary impact. In principle, drug abuse could lead either to increases or to decreases in welfare costs (because some people who die prematurely would otherwise be welfare recipients).

Data requirements and special considerations in developing countries

5

The International Guidelines present a methodology that nations may use to prepare estimates of the social costs of substance abuse. The application of the methodology, however, requires extensive data and information that many countries may not possess. There is strong interest in many nations, including developing nations, in understanding the nature and extent of the drug problem in all of its manifestations. For example, the 34 nations of the Western Hemisphere of the Americas have agreed to develop estimates of the social costs of substance abuse as part of the Organization of American States Multi-Evaluation Mechanism. International organizations like the WHO, UNDCP, and the EMCDDA are also participating in efforts to develop such estimates. While the methodological approach provides

The International Guidelines present a methodology that all nations may use to prepare estimates of the social costs of substance abuse. The application of the methodology, however, requires extensive data and information that many countries may not posses.

There is strong interest in many nations, including developing nations, in understanding the nature and extent of the drug problem in all of its manifestations. For example, the 34 nations of the Western Hemisphere of the Americas have agreed to develop estimates of the social costs of substance abuse as part of the Organization of American States Multi-Evaluation Mechanism. International organizations like the WHO, UNDCP, and the EMCDDA are also participating in efforts to develop such estimates. While the methodological approach provides a consistent framework for all nations to use, its application will be subject to tremendous variation due to cross-national data differences. Further confounding the successful application of the methodology is the fact that developing economies may have more difficulty using the methodology because of problems with their data infrastructure.

The application of the methodology is challenging. The estimate of social costs is developed through a series of sub-estimates, each requiring specific data that all nations may not posses. As is highlighted below, data are required about the incidence and prevalence of substance abuse, rates of addiction, mortality and morbidity, crime costs, health costs, and so forth. The problem of data availability raises a concern about the veracity of estimates when many of these data sources are unavailable.

Developing countries are likely to face even more of a challenge in applying the methodology to estimate the social costs of substance abuse due to gaps in data. Decisions about investments in data infrastructure will likely take a back seat to more urgent social and economic needs. Such economies may need direction in developing long-term strategies to select data systems that are within their means and best serve the needs of the methodology for estimating social costs. Developing countries may choose to selectively invest in data systems, hopefully procuring those data systems that offer the greatest advantages to the application of the methodology. Over the shorter term, developing countries will require other remedies to close the data gap for purposes of applying the methodology. These remedies range from setting the sub-estimate to zero (i.e., assume no cost attribution for the particular cost category), adopting estimates from external sources such as the experience of other nations in similar circumstances, to using rapid assessment methodologies. Where there is clearly insufficient data to conduct a COI study, another option is to undertake studies to estimate Disability Adjusted Life Years (DALYs) or Quality Adjusted Life Years (QALYs), thereby providing an epidemiological rather than an economic assessment of the burden of disease.

5.1 Data requirements for estimating social costs

The first question that any nation must address once it decides to estimate the social costs of substance abuse is whether data are available in sufficient quantity to apply the methodology to produce robust estimates of the major categories of costs associated with drug abuse. A tentative list of the data required to carry out a cost estimation study is as follows:

- Data on population structure by age and gender, and life expectancy by age and gender.
- Data required to estimate morbidity and mortality: prevalence data on drug use and injection drug use; number of deaths and hospitalizations, ideally by cause, age and gender; list of conditions which epidemiological research have shown to be attributable to drug use and the associated relative risks; estimates of the attributable fractions for certain causes of death and disease, based on local information, e.g., motor vehicle accidents, assaults, homicide, suicide.
- Health care costs: hospitalization costs, physician fees, costs of other professional services, and number of cases seen by physicians and other professional service providers by age and gender; ambulance costs (total costs, total number of trips, number of trips for drug-related causes);

costs of pharmaceuticals used to treat drug-related conditions (total number of prescriptions, number of prescriptions by cause).
- Policy costs: police, court and corrections costs; expenditures on prevention and research related to drugs; costs of training for physicians, nurses other health professionals, law enforcement.
- Costs of Employee Assistance Programmes and estimates of the proportion of such costs attributable to drugs.
- Indirect productivity costs: mean income by age and gender (to estimate morbidity costs) and present value of lifetime earnings by age and gender (to estimate costs of premature mortality).

The key issues for each of these data domains are whether data are available, in what form and from what source. Hopefully, some of these data will be collected from national censuses, surveys, or special population studies. In some cases, the information may not be available from formal surveys, but may be available in administrative records. Making estimates of such costs depends on gaining access to these data. The analytic challenge is to obtain data that will provide a plausible basis for attributing some proportion of the costs associated with the particular negative consequence to drug abuse. In other cases, data may not be available from any source. In such cases, a nation may wish to engage the use of rapid assessment methodologies or other means to fill the information gap.

5.2 Closing the data gap

In an ideal world, the data required to apply the methodology for estimating the social costs of substance abuse would be available to every nation. In reality, few nations possess such a wealth of data, which means that short-term solutions will be required.

One approach gaining popularity is the use of rapid assessment tools being developed by the WHO and other international agencies to gather data in particular topical areas. Another approach is to conduct special evaluations to provide plausible estimates of a component of the calculation of social costs. This is particularly useful to the challenge of attributing some proportion of the costs associated with the particular negative consequence to drug abuse (the attribution factor).

For some categories of social costs, a nation may be unable to obtain any information from any internal source. Rather than ignore the calculation of a sub-estimate, they may seek information for sub-estimates from external sources, defined here to represent information from other nations with similar situations or problems. External information can provide reasonable estimates of categories of costs while a longer-term data strategy is implemented. For example, until internal studies are available, it may be better to use the proportion of crime attributable to substance abuse in another (preferably, similar) country rather than ignore a potentially important cost element.

Interpretation of cost estimates and the relevance to evaluation of policies and programmes

Evaluation of policies and programs designed to reduce substance abuse is essential to inform public policy. There is a tendency to give considerable attention to the aggregate total cost estimates in COI studies. While the bottom-line figures are useful for setting policy agendas, it was noted earlier (see Section 1.2) that this is but one of several purposes to cost estimation studies. Equally important is economic evaluation, to ensure that resources are used appropriately. The estimation of the economic and social costs of substance abuse provides tools for economic evaluation of policies and programs.

It was noted earlier in Section 2.6 that the interpretation of cost estimate results depends in part on whether productivity losses are estimated using a human capital or a demographic approach as these two approaches are intended to address somewhat different research questions. In either case, aggregate estimates of the social costs of substance abuse are *not* designed to indicate the benefits that would be realised by effective prevention and harm reduction programs since:

- Some of these costs relate to past substance abuse (for example, smoking-attributable morbidity). These are, therefore, unavoidable costs.
- It would be unrealistic to expect the complete elimination of the abuse of any particular substance. Even for periods well into the future, when the effects of past abuse have washed out of the system, it may be possible to reduce the costs of substance abuse but certainly not to eliminate them completely.

Thus it is necessary to estimate the avoidable costs of substance abuse, in order to be able to indicate the extent of potential returns to harm minimisation programs. However, estimates of avoidable costs fail to indicate how these cost reductions might be achieved or whether the social benefits resulting from these programs would exceed their social costs. These issues can only be settled by a process of project appraisal.

Project appraisal evaluates the efficiency of alternative projects or alternative policies. Its aims are to determine, by a process of enumeration of the benefits and costs of alternative projects or policies, the appropriate level of public resources to be devoted to the problem and the particular solutions to which those resources should be devoted. Its objective is to maximise the social rate of return resulting from the use of public resources so that these resources can be used as efficiently as possible.

The viewpoint from which project appraisal is approached is that of the community as a whole, not of individuals, firms or the public sector. This social perspective complicates the analysis substantially since private project appraisal avoids many of the theoretical and practical difficulties that social appraisers must confront, valuation of benefits and choice of discount rate being two of the most important. Furthermore, since the viewpoint is that of the community as a whole, not just of the government, the issues are much more complex than those of public expenditure funding and public revenue benefits.

In principle, the process of project appraisal should lead to the allocation of resources to programs that yield at least a minimum test rate of return. This rate of return should take account of rates of return, calculated on a consistent basis, on investment in the private sector in order to ensure an efficient allocation of resources between private and public sectors. In practice, there are many types of public goods and services that the private sector is unlikely to ever supply (unless through private provision facilitated by public funding). Even if it were possible to calculate public and private rates of return on this consistent basis, there are political constraints on public expenditure levels. Consequently, the objective of project appraisal is usually to achieve the efficient allocation of previously determined public expenditure levels between competing public sector uses. Governments generally purport to be attempting to reduce the size of the public sector, on the grounds that private expenditures are more efficient than public expenditures. At this level of evaluation the appropriate evaluation tool is benefit-cost analysis (BCA).

The scope of project appraisal can be extended into program budgeting, which is a system of managing government expenditures by attempting to compare the program proposals of all government agencies authorised to achieve similar objectives (Hyman, 1996).

In many cases the objectives of public expenditure analysis may be even more modest. The objective of the evaluation exercise may be predetermined (for example, a reduction of ten per cent in juvenile smoking prevalence) so that the analysis is reduced to cost comparisons of alternative programs designed to achieve the same objective. In other situations it may be considered that it is so difficult to value a program's output so that BCA is impossible. In these circumstances cost-effectiveness analysis (CEA) is appropriate. A disadvantage of COI studies is that the results are not easily linked to the outcome of interventions. Even a state-of-the-art COI study does not provide an adequate basis for resource allocation. The WHO has produced resource documents on CEA that can assist in linking the costs of health care interventions to summary measures of population health outcomes such as DALYs (see, e.g., Murray et al., 2000).

CEA can be defined as a detailed comparison of the costs of alternative techniques for achieving the same predetermined objective. In practice, CEA can be used to determine how a given objective can be achieved at least cost or how a desired output can be maximised for a given cost. The objectives and the outputs of programs subject to CEA are almost always one-dimensional since, if alternative programs yield multiple outputs in different ratios, it becomes necessary to assign values to each type of output.

The advantage of CEA in its usual, more limited sense is that there is no need to value output benefits. This makes the analysis much simpler than BCA since it is necessary to identify only the costs of alternative interventions. This is generally a much more straightforward process than valuation of program benefits, even though significant problems may arise in the allocation of overhead costs.

The major disadvantage of CEA is that the policy objective is predetermined rather than arising from the analysis. CEA in itself is of no assistance in determining policy objectives. As has been noted by others, there is an assumption of CEA, rarely discussed, that the required additional resources need to be transferred from another health intervention or other sources.

A further extension of evaluation techniques comes in the form of cost-utility analysis (CUA). While CUA is the least common of the methods of economic evaluation identified, its use within the healthcare sector warrants some discussion. Cost utility analysis calculates the cost per specified health effect (of a program, a technology or a pharmacological intervention) and expresses outcomes as uniform units of health. These units are presumed to have similar values across all conditions. The health effects are weighted to reflect individual or societal preferences for different health outcomes.

The most common weighting units are Quality Adjusted Life Years (QALYs) and Disability Adjusted Life Years (DALYs) (Murray and Lopez, 1996). The QALY attempts to compare treatment priorities by identifying and measuring the utility of using resources to treat people of different health status, with different likely outcomes from treatment. A QALY is treated as a "Unit" of health which combines extension of life with a measure of its worth. Its use is particularly focussed on societal decisions relating to which good or service to produce relative to one another, i.e. allocative efficiency. There have been a number of "league tables" developed comparing QALY measures of quality and quantity of life years gained. For example it is thus possible to compare QALYS from resources spent on smoking cessation programs with resources spent on organ transplantation.

The DALY is a measure which combines healthy life years lost because of premature mortality with healthy life years lost because of disability. This measure is a useful economic tool as the resource implications of each component of the DALY can be identified and estimated. The total loss of DALYs, worldwide, reflects the global burden of disease.

CUA can be considered as a special form of cost-effectiveness analysis, in which "effects" are measured in health status, and can contribute to societal decision-making in its identification of allocative efficiency. While it is still a matter contention whether QALYs and DALYs can be effective and acceptable public policy tools, they are increasingly being used to contribute to economic evaluation in the health care sector.

Social benefit/cost analysis attempts to describe and quantify the social benefits and costs of a policy or program expressed in terms of a common monetary unit. The current value of the flow of social benefits over the life of a project is compared with the current value of the flow of expenditures which have yielded those benefits. Discounting techniques are used to permit comparison of the current values of differential flows over time of the benefits and expenditures. The costs and benefits, once valued in comparable terms, are then compared in terms of some criterion – a benefit/cost ratio or some measure of the project's rate of return.

Aggregate substance abuse cost exercises should identify and place values on all the costs of abuse of the substance under review. Any reduction of these costs due to the implementation of a particular program will represent benefits of that program. Thus, the theoretical and practical issues involved in the valuation of program benefits should already have been faced in the substance abuse cost study. A human capital-based approach should provide all the necessary information, including discounted future costs. The demographic-based approach will not directly yield information about future substance abuse costs, so that extra analysis will be necessary.

Aggregate abuse cost estimates should already have made the necessary distinctions between private and social costs and should also have ensured that double counting of costs has been avoided by including only real (not pecuniary) costs. The estimates should already have taken account of valuation problems including the impact of private market imperfections, such as monopoly power or managed exchange rate regimes, and the difficulties of placing valuations on intangibles such as pain, other forms of suffering and loss of life. (For a review of issues involved in estimating the costs of tobacco use see Lightwood, Collins, Lapsley and Novotny, 2000.)

FIGURE 5 – INTERPRETATION OF SUBSTANCE ABUSE COST ESTIMATES

Type of estimate	Interpretation of results	Example of policy use
Aggregate costs	Total external costs of substance abuse compared with the alternative situation of no substance abuse	Indication of the size of the substance abuse problem
Avoidable costs	Potential economic benefits from substance abuse harm minimisation strategies	Determination of the appropriate level of resources to be devoted to harm minimisation strategies
Costs incidence	The distribution of the external costs of substance abuse among various community groupings	Mobilisation of support from various groups (for example, the business community) for anti-substance abuse programs
Disaggregated costs	External costs of substance abuse disaggregated by categories	Economic evaluation (cost-benefit or cost-effectiveness analysis) of harm minimisation programs
Budgetary impact	The impact of substance abuse on government expenditures and revenues	Assessment of the case for industry compensation payments to government as a result of excessive use of substances which the industry produces

Source: adapted from Collins and Lapsley (1998)

Figure 5 presents a summary of the different types of costs which can be identified within a costing study, and the ways in which the results can be interpreted. The disaggregated costs provide essential tools for further types of economic evaluation including those identified in this chapter.

Summary and conclusions

This document has presented proposed guidelines for estimating the economic costs associated with substance abuse. The purpose of these guidelines is to improve the validity and comparability of cost estimates in different societies. The development of improved cost estimates also offers the potential to develop more complete cost-benefit analyses of policies and programmes aimed at reducing the harm associated with the use of psychoactive substances.

A general framework has been proposed for the development of cost estimates. It has been argued that economic cost studies should be conducted within the framework of cost-of-illness studies. In cost estimation studies, the impact of substance abuse on the material welfare of a society is estimated by examining the social costs of treatment, prevention, research, law enforcement and lost productivity plus some measure of the quality of life years lost. It is recognized that data are frequently lacking for many of these costs.

However, in many countries it will be possible to develop reasonable estimates for some, if not most, of the costs associated with substance abuse. Thus, these guidelines should be viewed as a framework rather than a rigorous methodology to be applied in every situation.

An intriguing possibility is the development of special "satellite accounts" in the System of National Accounts (SNA) to estimate the costs of substance abuse. In 1993 those concerned with defining the SNA framework issued a new manual, which included the concept of satellite accounts.[15] Its Chapter 11 sets down criteria for satellite analysis and accounts. Their initial concern is better representing the physical environment in the SNA, but they will also be used for characterizing the behaviour of non-market activities, such as housework. It would also seem a sensible development in COI studies in general, and those involving substance abuse in particular, to develop them in a satellite SNA account framework, as far as that is possible.

Appendix A: Glossary of common terms used in economic cost studies[17]

Each discipline has its own terminology. In a growing interdisciplinary area as is the evaluation of substance abuse, such terminology, while necessary, can be a hindrance. The following glossary is of terms which have come up in the course of the work thus far. The glossary is confined to terms used in the various papers and does not claim to be comprehensive, or to replace more extensive dictionaries of health economics.

Wherever possible a standard dictionary term is used. Where there are a variety of definitions we have used the one which corresponds most closely to that in the papers.

In some cases where the term is relatively new and/or contentious, or will be unfamiliar to the non-specialist economist, there is some elaboration of its meaning. We have clustered some common terms, often opposites, together so the reader can gain a better idea of the distinction or contrast that is being sought. Words in bold in the text have their own reference.

Brian Easton and Robert Bowie

abuse see **use**

addiction & dependence
can be treated as synonymous in the case of drugs/substances. Addiction is defined by Jacob and Fehr a "a state of dependence upon a drug substance which is harmful to physical or mental health, social wellbeing, and/or economic functioning". This poses a problem for economists as to what extent the phenomenon involves irrationality.

aetiologic fraction or **attributable fraction**
refers the proportion of cases of a disorder (cause of disease or death, or a particular type of crime) that can be causally attributed to a particular risk factor, such as drug misuse.

avoidable costs & unavoidable costs
In the context of cost-of-illness studies avoidable costs are those which could be avoided in the future if the appropriate treatment or policy were to be implemented. However some costs are the result of actions taken in the past, and are unavoidable, despite the new treatment or policy. If everyone stopped smoking, there would still be morbidity and mortality effects from the physiological damage of past smoking. The continuing costs of these would be unavoidable. Avoidability depends in part on the time period under consideration – the longer the time period, the greater the proportion of costs which are avoidable.

benefit cost analysis see **cost-benefit analysis**

benefits see **costs**

budgetary impact studies estimate the economic costs and benefits of substance use and misuse to government budgets through its outlays and revenues. Care needs to be taken to clearly define "government", since it may refer to the national government only or include lower levels of government such as states and local authorities.

consensual crimes see **victimless crimes**

consequences/causality/costs is a summary of the three-step process in the Harwood paper for the framework for cost-of-illness studies. The elaboration is

– identify the tangible consequences attributable to substance abuse;
– document causality between substance abuse and the consequences, and quantify frequency;
– assign economic values.

Maynard et al use a parallel identification/measurement/valuation framework.

consumer surplus is the difference between what consumers would be willing to pay for a good or service and the market price that they are actually required to pay.

core & non-core. Core costs in relation to substance abuse are those which occur primarily within the domain of the health system, while non-core costs occur outside it. The public health sector is a part of the core, but so is the private health sector. See institutional arrangements.

cost-benefit, cost-effectiveness analyses, and cost utility analysis. Cost-benefit analysis (CBA), also known as **benefit-cost analysis**, involves the enumeration and evaluation in terms of a common unit, usually money, of all opportunity costs and benefits of taking a particular action. The costs and benefits are measured from the societal viewpoint, and usually ignore the distribution within the nation. If the benefit of an action exceeds the costs then there is a sense in which it is in the interests of the nation to take that course. Where there are costs and benefits occurring through time, the method involves discounting. **Cost-effectiveness analysis** (CEA) is the procedure for identifying the least-cost means of pursuing a particular objective. For instance there may be two (or more) treatment alternatives. A CEA would evaluate which treatment produced the given outcome using least resources. **Cost utility analysis** (CUA) calculates the cost per specified health effect (of a program, a technology or a pharmaceutical intervention) and expresses outcomes as uniform units of health. These units are presumed to have similar values across all conditions.

cost-effectiveness analysis see **cost-benefit analysis**

cost-of-illness analysis (COI) asks what are the total costs incurred by a particular illness. Since the cost measure is an **opportunity cost,** they in effect ask what would be the resources released to society if the illness did not exist. Thus the cost-of-illness is related to the benefits in a **cost-benefit analysis.** The economic and social costs of substance abuse are a cost-of-illness analysis.

costs, opportunity costs, historical costs, & benefits. Opportunity cost is the value of a resource in its most highly valued alternative use. It is the concept economists use when valuing costs. They ask if a resource is not used for this purpose what is its value in the next best purpose. In a competitive market in which all goods are traded and where there are no market imperfections, the opportunity cost of a resource is revealed by its market price. However these assumptions do not always hold, as when the resource is not bought and sold – it is non-market. Sometimes payments which appear to a layperson to be costs are not opportunity costs, and are left out of the calculations or calculated in a different way. e.g. historical costs and transfers. **Historical costs** reflect the past payments for a resource, but they may not represent the opportunity cost. If some medical equipment it is now useless, its opportunity cost is zero or the scrap value, while its historical cost is the cost of purchase, less depreciation. Benefits are the gains, before costs are deducted, of any particular course of action, preventive program, therapy, treatment, etc. They are usually valued in money terms. Ideally the valuation is **willingness to pay.**

cost utility analysis see **cost benefit analysis**

counterfactual propositions are the situation which the economist sets up as the alternative to the current one in order to assess the benefits and opportunity costs (e.g. for a cost-benefit analysis) of a different policy, treatment or circumstance. For instance the economist may be investigating the policy of raising taxes on alcohol, or of a new treatment regime for a narcotic, or the situation in which tobacco had never been available. Cost-of-illness studies have the counterfactual proposition that the illness does not occur. There may be more than one counterfactual proposition to a situation, so the results may be very sensitive to the exact assumption. For instance, it could be argued that the counterfactual to a situation without alcohol is greater use of narcotics.

DALYs (disability adjusted life years) see **QALYs**

demographic approach & human capital approach. The demographic approach (Collins and Lapsley, 1991) involves the **counterfactual proposition** of what would have occurred to the population if the illness (or whatever) had never occurred in the past. It is essentially a **retrospec-**

tive approach, and reflects a **national accounting** method. The **human capital approach** used extensively in cost-benefit analyses (Harwood, 1994) involves tracing the future effects of the change in policy (or whatever) on the population. Its counterfactual proposition is about what would happen if the illness ceased from the present, and values future gains by **discounting** to the present. It is essentially a **prospective** approach.

dependence see **addiction**

direct costs & indirect costs. In health economics **direct costs** are usually the costs to the **core** health system. **Indirect costs** are those incurred elsewhere, notably but not exclusively **productivity lost.** However elsewhere in economics the terms refer to variable costs and fixed costs respectively, and these (or other) definitions sometimes are used in health economics.

disability adjusted life years (DALYs) see **QALYs.**

discount rate see **discounting**

discounting, discount rate, & present value
Discounting is the procedure by which a flow of benefits or costs incurred or accruing at different points in time is expressed as an equivalent money sum at a single point in time, normally the present. It is especially important where there is an investment element to the activity. Discounting involves the use of a **discount rate,** which is difficult to measure or agree upon. In principle the discount rate is the rate of exchange between money sums at different times, in effect an interest rate. In the case where the sum is discounted back to the current date, it is called the **present value.**

double counting, insurance. Double counting, the phenomenon where a resource is included in a total more than once, needs to be avoided. For example **insurance** spending has to be split into two components. The first is the actual cost of administering the scheme, the **transaction cost.** The second is the payment to the insured. This benefit is offset by the cost in the insurance payment. It would be double counting to include the insurance payment (except for the transaction costs) such as for motor vehicle coverage, and also the cost incurred by the payment the insurance covered, such as the cost of car repairs.

equilibrium. In the context of these studies, **equilibrium** is the situation where there has been full adjustment to a changed external factor (often arising out of a difference in the **counterfactual scenario**). In **partial equilibrium** analysis, the changes only occur in an isolated part of the economy (usually a market) but do not impact significantly on an economy as a whole. This is the usual assumption in costs of substance abuse studies. However where the market or industry is sufficiently large and there are significant feedback effects on the economy as a whole, the analysis has to be based on a **general equilibrium** approach. Examples in substance abuse might involve a drug producing industry which was a sizeable part of the economy as a whole (or its export sector).

external costs see **internal costs**

general equilibrium see **equilibrium**

gross costs & net costs. Gross costs consist of all costs, and ignore any offsetting **benefits.** If the benefits are deducted the remainder are net costs. In the event of a net cost being negative (i.e. benefits exceeding gross costs), there is a net benefit.

GDP see **gross domestic product**

GNP see **gross domestic product**

gross national product see **gross domestic product**

gross domestic product (GDP) is the total money value of all the final goods and services produced in the economy in a period (usually a year). Typically it covers only those activities which occur in the market (including the government sectors, although there are some minor exceptions. **Gross nation product (GNP)** is GDP plus the net property income from abroad. The fundamental distinction is that GDP covers the economic activities within a nation's boundaries, while GNP refers to the activities which the nation's people are involved with. They differ (but usually not by much in quantitative terms) because nationals own some production which occurs abroad, and some of the domestic (within national boundaries) production is owned by foreigners. The **SNA** and international agencies such as the OECD concentrate on GDP, but some countries, notably the USA pay more attention to GNP.

human capital approach see **demographic approach**

identification/measurement/valuation is the summary of the three step process used in **costs of illness** studies (Maynard et al., 1994). The elaboration is

- which elements to include in the work;
- how to measure the effects in each area over the relevant time period;
- how to value these effects in a common unit of account.

Harwood (1994) uses the parallel **consequence/causality/cost** framework.

illicit drugs & licit drugs. It is usually unlawful to possess or use **illicit drugs,** which typically include narcotics. **Licit** drugs are those whose use is generally lawful, and usually include alcohol and tobacco (although in some countries alcohol consumption is unlawful). Note that it is possible to misuse a licit drug, as occurs with some prescription drugs.

incidence prevalence & point prevalence.
Incidence is the number of instances of illness commencing, or of persons falling ill, during a given period for a population. It is about new events. **Prevalence** is the number of instances of a given disease or other condition in a given population at a designated time. If the period is not mentioned, the concept usually refers to the situation at a specified point in time, that is **point prevalence.**

indirect costs see **direct costs**

insurance (treatment of) see **double counting**

intangible costs see tangible costs

internal costs & external costs. Economists usually assume that individuals make decisions in their own interests. The costs and benefits taken into account are **internalized** while those which are ignored are **external** to the decision. These externalities occur when the individuals making decisions ignore the consequences of their decisions for others. A complication is that while internal costs are **private** costs to the decision-maker, some of the external costs may be private costs to others. The complement of private cost in the context of these studies is **social** cost, some of which may be in the private sector.

irrational see **rational**

licit drugs see **illicit drug**

marginal is the term economists use when they are considering the effects of one extra unit. Thus marginal cost is the additional costs from the extra unit, and marginal value is the extra value. If the marginal value exceeds the marginal cost it makes sense to use the unit, and to repeat this for the next unit until the net marginal gain is zero.

marginal cost see **marginal**

marginal value see **marginal**

market & non-market. The point of this distinction is to observe that while many **costs** and **benefits** occur **tangibly** in the market others, of sometimes greater importance, occur outside it. This includes **intangibles** but also activities in the household and elsewhere such as carework and housework, which are not paid, but nevertheless involves the resource of labour effort (and which may be diverted from the market).

morbidity is any subjective or objective departure from a state of physiological or psychological well-being. (Sickness, illness, and morbid condition are synonyms in this sense.)

mortality refers to death.

national accounts are a system of analysis the production, distribution, expenditure, and financing of a nation. In recent years the international standards have been extended from a primary concern on **market** activities, to cover **non-market** ones such as the environment and housework. Some features of **cost-of-illness** studies can be seen to be in a national accounting framework.

net costs see **gross costs**

opportunity costs see **benefits**

partial equilibrium see **equilibrium**

point prevalence see **incidence**

present value see **discounting**

prevalence see **incidence**

private, public, and social costs. Private costs have two meanings in the economics literature. They may refer to the costs considered by the single private decision maker **(internal costs)**, or they may refer to the costs of those in the private sector, not carried by the public sector. As a rule **public costs** refer to costs in the public (i.e. government) sector. The complement of private costs in the first sense of the private decision maker is usually **social costs**. Because there is no uniformity of definition, the terms "public" and "private" should always be treated with care.

productivity loss. As a result of illness a person may be less productive because of higher absenteeism or lower output on the job. This loss of production is included in the **costs of illness**. In principle loss of productivity should cover consequences outside the **market** economy, such as reductions in human carework and housework by the sick person.

project appraisal evaluates the efficiency of alternative projects or alternative policies. Its aims are to determine, by a process of enumeration of the benefits and costs of alternative projects or policies, the appropriate level of public resources to be devoted to the problem and the particular solutions to which those resources should be devoted. It helps to maximise the social rate of return resulting from the use of public resources by identifying the most efficient use for these resources.

prospective & retrospective. A **retrospective** analysis typically involves a **counterfactual** proposition about an event which might have occurred in the past as it impacts on the situation today, whereas a **prospective** analysis asks about the effects of a counterfactual event with effects which begin at the point in time of the analysis (or shortly after) and with consequences into the future.

public costs see **private costs**

QALYs, or **quality adjusted life years,** sometimes used in **CEAs,** measure any years of life gained from a treatment adjusted for consequential changes in the quality of the life as the result of an improvement in the enjoyment of the years from reduced pain, increased mobility, and so forth. **DALYs,** or **disability adjusted life years,** are another way of measuring changes in the quality of life.

quality adjusted life years see **QALYs**

quantifiable & non-quantifiable. Many benefits and costs are directly **quantifiable** (or measurable), or can be indirectly quantified. However in the case of some of the most important – often **social** – ones, it is not possible to do so, and these are called **non-quantifiable.** Sometimes ad hoc methods are used to put estimates on non-quantifiable costs, rather than leave them out of the evaluation altogether.

rapid assessment methods are being developed by the WHO and other international agencies to enable data-poor countries to be able to make a broad assessment of the likely importance of a policy, or the need to gather more information, using data which are likely to be available but may not be comprehensive or particularly accurate.

rational, non-rational & irrational. Economics assumes that individuals are generally **rational,** pursuing their own best interests as best they can. ("Bounded" rationality recognizes they may not have the information, time, or best decision strategies to do so – that decision making involves costs.) Note that the **internal** decision may ignore the **external** costs to others. However the existence of **addiction** and **drug abuse** may suggest that sometimes individuals act **irrationally,** failing to pursue their own best interests, even in a bounded way. Collins and Lapsley explore this issue further in the section on addictive and non-addictive consumption. Their conclusion is that where drug consumption is irrational, the expenditure on the drugs is not a benefit to the individual and hence is a part of the total costs of abuse.

risk factor refers to a characteristics of an individual or the environment which is associated with an increased risk of a particular disorder.

retrospective see **prospective**

SNA, the System of National Accounts, is the international standard for measuring GDP

social costs see **internal costs and private costs**

structural unemployment see **workforce**

system of national accounts see **SNA**

tangible & intangible. Tangible costs and benefits are those which can be easily measured in money terms. **Intangible** ones cannot be so easily measured, although it is often useful to make an attempt to do so (perhaps using a **willingness to pay** approach). Very often the intangible costs involving changes in quality and length of life prove to be more important in the valuation than the tangible ones.

transfers or transfer payments (such taxes, subsidies, and welfare payments) do not relate to resource costs, so that the cost to one person is exactly offset by the benefit to someone else (as when somebody's tax is another's social security payment). It would be **double counting** to include the transfer payment as a cost, but not to offset the contribution. Again **transaction costs** may be relevant.

transaction costs are those costs involved in a transaction. They include any costs for administering the transaction (e.g. the government and private compliance costs of the tax system), plus any losses from behavioural responses (as when taxpayers reduce effort because of higher tax rates). The past practice has been to assume transaction costs may be neglected because they are small. They may not be.

unavoidable costs see **avoidable costs**

unemployment see **workforce**

use & abuse. Economists tend not to judge the usefulness of the **use** of a product or substance to the user, other than in terms of the user's assessment. However the existence of **addiction** and **irrational behaviour** would seem to undermine that assumption. Other disciplines seem not to have a rigorous definition of **abuse.** A medical definition might be "drug abuse is deemed to occur when a relevant aetiologic fraction is greater than zero, i.e. when drug abuse adversely affects the health of the user". Economists tend to assume that a rational user takes this detriment into consideration when they are making the use decision. Sometimes the term is used pejoratively. Abel's *Dictionary of Alcohol Use and Abuse* (1985) remarks, no doubt ironically, that alcohol abuse is "consumption to the point where it results in social disapproval", which is the sort of judgement that economists' try to avoid. Even so the term may be used as a short-hand for some longer concept which is carefully defined. For instance Collins and Lapsley define the term in their paper as "when the use of a drug or substance imposes social [external] costs in addition to private [internal] costs", and devote an entire section to refining their definition.

value of life recognises that the effect of a treatment (or policy) may be to save lives, and that this effect should be included in a **cost-benefit analysis.** Otherwise the analysis would ignore life enhancing treatments, and comparisons would favour those which made no such comparisons. On the other hand the notion of putting a finite sum on the "value of life" might seem offensive. To put an infinite sum, however, would mean that there could be no trade-off for improvements in the quality of life. For example a CBA would be likely to favour a zero speed limit for cars if the value of life was infinite. The study's approach has favoured the replacement of a value of life concept with a **social gains from additional life years.** Whichever concept is used, it is difficult to get an agreed value for the item. A description of approaches for estimating the value of life will be found in the Maynard et al paper.

value theory explains how prices are determined. ("Value" was often used in the nineteenth century as meaning long run prices). It is a central part of the modern economics paradigm and underpins the **system of national accounting (SNA)** and **cost-benefit analysis.**

victimless crimes. Certain types of crime involve no apparent "victim" and are sometimes termed **consensual** or victimless crimes. These are activities such as sex for pay, illegal gambling and the illegal drug trade. In some nations it is not uncommon to find some drug dependent persons in these professions.

willingness to pay is a measure of benefit opportunity cost, especially where an **intangible is** involved. Measurement can involve polling individuals, asking what they would be prepared to pay for the resource or outcome. There is a growing body of empirical studies – such as using surveys – which attempt to measure the willingness to pay.

workforce is the term used to cover that part of the labour force which is in active paid employment, and is not unemployed. While the conventional division is between the labour force (which covers the workforce, and those who are unemployed) and not-in-the-labour force, only those employed in the workforce directly cause a loss of (market) production through a loss of employment effectiveness as a result of poorer health. The **unemployed** are those who are not employed but actively seeking paid employment. The **structurally unemployed** are those unemployed who tend not have the skills demanded by employers. Thus if an employed person leaves the workforce (say through illness or death) the employer is unlikely to turn to a structurally unemployed person to fill the vacancy.

Appendix B: The evaluation of economies with significant drug production industries

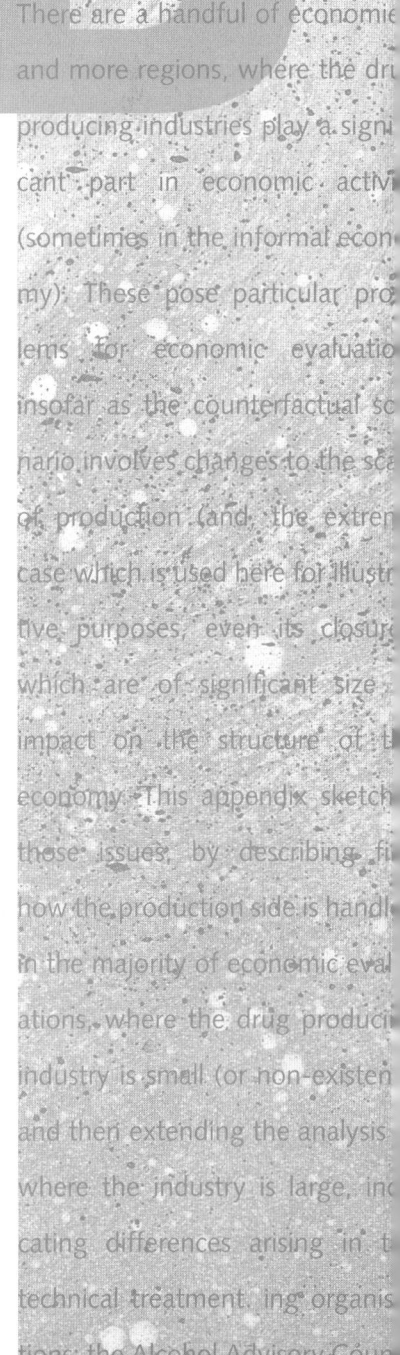

There are a handful of economies, and more regions, where the drug producing industries play a significant part in economic activity (sometimes in the informal economy). These pose particular problems for economic evaluation, insofar as the counterfactual scenario involves changes to the scale of production (and, the extreme case which is used here for illustrative purposes, even its closure), which are of significant size to impact on the structure of the economy. This appendix sketches those issues, by describing first how the production side is handled in the majority of economic evaluations, where the drug producing industry is small (or non-existent), and then extending the analysis to where the industry is large, indicating differences arising in the technical treatment.

It should be emphasized that the fundamental analysis is exactly the same for both cases. The differences arise because in the small industry case there are some acceptable simplifying analytic assumptions – in technical terms "partial equilibrium" analysis may be used instead of "general equilibrium" analysis. It should also be clear from the following account that there is no simple line between "large" and "small". The distinction is whether the simplifications are justified. This is usually a straightforward judgement in the case of whole economies, but may be more ambiguous in the case of regions. It should also be noted that the drug production industry may be functioning legally or illegally (usually depending upon whether its output is licit or illicit), which also affects the evaluation, as is discussed below.

The distinctions of a drug producing industry being either large or small in the economy and of its activities being legal or illegal, generates a two by two table, as follows (with an example in each of the four countries).

	Small industry	Large industry
Legal production	Tobacco in Virginia	Tobacco in Zimbabwe
Illegal production	Cannabis in New Zealand	Cocaine in Colombia

As always, the counterfactual assumption is crucial in setting out the cost evaluation. There is a wide range of possible scenarios which will reflect particular circumstances. For instance, the small-illegal counterfactual is likely to be a consequence of the assumption that local or national drug consumption ends. In the case of the small-legal industry the elimination of local consumption is unlikely to end the industry and it will turn to (or increase) exporting (unless it is heavily protected and inefficient). The large-legal industry is probably already a major exporter and its closure or reduction in scale may reflect some international shift, which has nothing to do with changes in local consumption. The possibilities of what might close down a large-illegal industry are varied, including a drop in world demand or effective supply control policies. The following discussion is based on a generic closure, but the particularities of the counterfactual may affect a specific estimate.

Relatively small-scale production of legal drugs

While a particular industry may be large in a region, this category covers those legal drug producing industries that are small in relation to the national economy as a whole. There will be transition effects, but it is usually assumed that in the medium to long run following industry closure (or reduction in scale) the factors of production (e.g., land, labour and capital) will be redeployed to the same extent they had in the past (or perhaps that currently unemployed factors will take up in their place). Depending on the degree of mobility, it is possible that some factors (e.g. labour) may migrate to other regions (in which case the social cost of the industry in the region may differ from the economy as a whole).

However, some of those production resources may be industry specific. This may apply most notably to land. The next best use of land currently used for drug production may be valued considerably less by the market. As far as measures of opportunity cost are concerned, the social loss from the industry equals the reduction in the market return for those specific factors. It does not equal the total value of the production resource. For example, suppose an industry was annually producing US$ 100 million worth of tobacco, and the next best alternative was potatoes with an output value of US$ 90 million. Then the social cost of closing the tobacco industry would be US$ 10 million per annum, not US$ 100 million per annum.

It cannot be understated that it is quite wrong to describe the gross output of an industry as its social cost of closure. The statement applies only if none of the resources used in the small-scale legal drug production could be deployed in any other economic activity. The economic cost is the difference between the returns to the factors of production of the industry and the returns to the next best option. This is a general economic proposition and does not just apply to drug producing industries.

Note that the counterfactual scenario may entail a complicated story of other industries adjusting. It does not assume that smokers simply switch to buying potatoes. So the estimated social cost is the net effect. However, because the industry is small, it is unnecessary to trace the impact of its closure on the economy as a whole. As a general rule, the long-term industry-specific resources used in a small-scale legal drug industry will be land and possibly some labour skills. While some capital may be industry-specific in the short run (e.g. drying kilns for tobacco), in the long run it will depreciate and be replaced by some other capital (e.g. warehouses for sorting potatoes).

The meaning of this estimate of the social cost of drug production is as follows. If the industry were to close down (or reduce in scale) there would be a loss of material welfare equal to the estimated social cost. However, this is in principle the same value as the loss of private consumer surplus if there is no excessive consumption. (In practice the two methods may treat second order effects differently, and of course there will be estimation errors.) The relative balance between the social costs of production and changes in consumer surplus arises because changes in production values are driven by changes in consumer values, and vice versa. It would be double counting to include the production and consumption losses in the aggregate, since they are two ways of measuring the same thing.

Where there is excessive consumption, the methodology discounts the apparent market value to consumers of that consumption. Thus the production value will exceed the estimated consumption value. This means that the production is that much less value to the economy. Production values exceed the value that the consumers use in their voluntary decisions. Again it would be double counting to add the change in production values to the changes in consumer surplus. Moreover, where there is excessive consumption, it would be an overestimate to use the production values in place of consumer values.

Relatively small-scale production of illegal drugs

The measurement of the social costs for small-scale illegal drug production will be similar to that for small-scale legal drug production, if the counterfactual scenario is the same. However, there are two relatively minor differences when illicit drug production is involved. First, when small-scale illegal drug production is curtailed, production resources may shift from the informal (unmeasured) economy to the formal measured one, and thus give a false impression of an increase in GDP. Attention should be drawn to any offsetting reduction in the informal economy. Second, depending on the precise assumptions, there may be a real gain to the economy if there is a reduction in policing and other related law enforcement costs.

A major difference may be that the illegal industry is avoiding tax. Its closure and replacement by legitimate industries would increase the tax base. This is a benefit to the economy insofar as other taxes can be reduced and the burden of taxation reduced.

The small-scale illegal drug production industry may also be associated with some corruption of the type we shall discuss in the large-illegal industry. However, the magnitude will be small, the consequences less endemic, and the evaluation of the impact on production and the public sector manageable.

This cost of closure is to be treated similarly to the similar estimates for the cost of closure for small-legal industries.

Relatively large-scale production of legal drugs

The fundamental difference between a large and small industry is that the closure or severe curtailment of a large industry could well have a marked impact on the economy as a whole, involving major adjustments. For instance, if an industry is a major exporter, if there is not any substantial external support such as international financial assistance and the next best use of production resources is much less remunerative, the closure of this industry would mean that the economy would experience a major loss of foreign exchange revenue, the real exchange rate would fall, there would be a marked reduction in real incomes, and the response would be major structural change in the long run. Indeed, it is conceivable that closure could result in a major depression in the short run.

Because of the size of the industry in the economy as a whole, it is not possible to use the special case of the "partial equilibrium" analysis underpinning the small industry approach. It is not necessary here to describe "general equilibrium" analysis, which is a well-established procedure for examining the long run impact of – among other things – industry closure. The result will be to give an estimated value of GDP while the industry is functioning, and compare this to the estimated value of the GDP after the industry is closed down or reduced substantially in scale. The difference (after adjusting for price changes) is loss of social welfare, or the social cost of closure or scale reduction. Note that the data requirements for general equilibrium analysis are substantial – considerably more than the national accounts which may be used for the partial equilibrium analysis. In practice many countries have insufficient data to use the technique.

To understand the significance of the estimated social cost of industry closure using a general equilibrium model, assume that there is zero local consumption, so that all the production is exported. In this case the reduction in GDP represents the actual loss of production and hence consumption and welfare to the country. This point also applies for a study from a regional perspective. (Insofar as there is a reduction in domestic consumption this needs to be allowed for in the interpretation).

The loss of welfare of the large-scale production of legal drugs in a particular country is offset (subject to second order effects) by the gains to the other countries whose consumers desist or reduce excessive consumption (assuming that is the counterfactual scenario). Thus the overall gains and losses will depend very much on the geographic unit used in the analysis. Where this is matter of significance – typically a large industry in an open economy, a comprehensive evaluation of costs should include estimates of the burden of costs to the rest of the world.

Relatively large-scale production of illegal drugs

If the industry under consideration involves illegal activities, the measurement difficulties increase. Almost certainly the quality of the economic data base for illegal activities is lower than for legal activities, and often substantially so. Among the major difficulties are:

- The industry is poorly measured;
- the industry generates other transfers and transactions which are poorly measured;
- where the industry interacts with the legal system the prices of the transactions may be poorly measured; and
- the industry is often in a developing economy with a low per capita income which has a limited data base anyway (see Chapter 5).

However, it is not only the lack of data for the general equilibrium model which limits the ability to calculation of social costs. Large illegal industries are almost certainly associated with pervasive and endemic corruption that it distorts civil society and good government. Among their effects are:

- The public sector is corrupted and functions inefficiently;
- there is institutional instability which generates commercial uncertainty and discourages legitimate investment (including overseas development investment) and encourages capital flight (including flight of highly trained human capital);
- enforcement, control, and elimination measures directed at the illicit drug production industry may have side effects such as environmental

damage from attempted crop controls which entail significant costs to the local economy;
- market prices may be distorted from true reflecting true social values; and
- there are costs to the economy from warring among the drug barons, and the drugs may maintain guerilla activities at a significant scale.

The counterfactual scenario is that without this industry the country would experience a stable society and good governance. The various collateral activities would not occur.

In principle it is possible to characterize in quantitative detail the society with and without the illegal industry. In practice it does not seem possible to do this, in a reasonably rigorous way.

It is likely that a general equilibrium analysis that focuses only on the production shifts – were it possible – would, as in the case of a large-scale legal drug production industry, show a decrease in material welfare if the large-scale illegal drug industry were closed or substantially scaled back. However, it is likely that the elimination of corruption in the governance of society would result in a net higher GDP. How much higher, we just do not know. The cost of closure for large-illegal industries seems appears likely to be negative (i.e., the net impact on GDP would be positive) but one cannot say with certainty until better data are available.

Appendix C: Comparing social costs of substance abuse to GDP

In Section 3.8, it was noted that one cannot, strictly speaking, compare estimates of the costs of substance abuse to the Gross Domestic Product (GDP) because the former include both tangible and intangible costs while GDP is generally limited to tangible outputs of the economy. The purpose of this brief appendix is to describe how it is possible to make meaningful comparisons of any tangible measure. It is recommended any comparison should be in two parts:

- the tangible social costs of substance abuse which assess the consequential loss of material output can be compared with US$ GDP (the dollar sign being included to confirm the variable is measured in monetary units). If the value of the tangible material costs is US$ T then the ratio US$ T/US$ GDP measures the effective increase in material goods and services available if the substance abuse were eliminated (or whatever is involved in the counterfactual scenario). (Where the tangible social costs include non-market production, the comparison is not quite consistent and either those non-market– but tangible– costs should be excluded, or GDP should be augmented by non-market production. The former is easier).
- the intangible costs of substance abuse which assess the loss or deterioration of live above that of any material cost should be compared with the same measure applied to the population a whole. We illustrate the principle when QALYs are being used. Suppose the consequential loss in QALYs from substance abuse are equal IT quality life years. If the value of one QALY is determined to be US$ V, then the calculated loss will be US$ V x IT = US$ VIT (say). Suppose the total QALYs in the existing population is P. Then its value will be US$ V x P = US$ VP (say). (The calculation of P may not be easy, as it involves an estimation of the average QALY per person, which will be less than unity because there is disability within the population not caused by substance abuse).

The ratio US$ VIT/US$ VP (or IT/P) measures the proportional increase in quality life years if there is no substance abuse (or whatever is the counterfactual scenario). This easily understood ratio is a meaningful measure of the impact of substance abuse on the quality of life. (If the calculations are based on deaths caused by substance abuse, then the denominator is total population, and the ratio an indicator of how much larger the population would be were there no substance abuse).

For comparison purposes then, we recommend that the social costs of substance abuse be presented as representing a US$ T/US$ GDP reduction in material welfare and an IT/P (= US$ VIT/US$ VP) reduction in quality life years. If an aggregate is required the sum US$ T + US$ VIT should be used, but it should NEVER be compared with GDP.

This approach resolves the issue for those who have an ethical objection to valuing human life. They can still report the two proportions, but need not report the aggregate, noting that the ratio IT/P need not include a valuation of life but is simply a comparison of (adjusted) life years or lives.

Since there is no internationally agreed procedure for measuring the intangible costs of life– in contrast to the well established, theoretically underpinned, internationally accepted measure GDP– then international comparisons of the costs of substance abuse which involve valuing life (above that of its contribution to material production) are unclear. (While valuation methodologies vary it is not obvious how to compare dollar values between countries even when the valuation methodology– such as willingness-to-pay– is the same).

Because the IT/P ratio is not dependent upon the dollar value of a human life (since it multiplies both the denominator and numerator) this helps resolve the problem of international comparisons. (It should be noted the ratio does not assume that a QALY or similar measure in country A has the same value as one in country B. At this stage in international comparisons it is probably useful to avoid such comparisons).

Even so the ratio is likely to depend on whether the evaluation is in QALYs, DALYs, lives or other measure. Moreover some of the differences in the method for calculating quantitative magnitude (e.g. QALY vs. DALY) will cancel out between the top and bottom measures of the ratio.

The comparison of tangible costs is relatively straightforward because the proportion of GDP is a useful (but, of course, incomplete) measure which is broadly comparable (although any rigorous comparison requires comparable counterfactual scenarios and similar methods of estimation).

Meanwhile the IT/P ratio has some merits for intangible cost comparisons. It is not dependent upon the dollar value for human lives and some of the differences in method cancel out because the same method is applied to the numerator and denominator.

We recommend this ratio as the best practical way of making international comparisons of the non-material costs of substance abuse, until there is more international agreement on a procedure. However, it is unlikely that it will ever make sense to compare intangible costs with GDP.

Appendix D: Application of the guidelines in cost estimation studies

The purpose of this appendix is to briefly illustrate the practical application of these guidelines. Since the publication of the first edition of the International Guidelines for Estimating the Costs of Substance Abuse, the guidelines have been used in several COI studies. Among its principal aims, the guidelines are intended to enhance consensus on appropriate methodology and promote greater comparability regarding the results of studies in different countries. In agreement, the authors of the guidelines used the guidelines in subsequent COI studies conducted in Australia, Canada, New Zealand and the U.S. (Collins and Lapsley, 1995; Collins and Lapsley, 1996; Easton, 1998; Single et al., 1998; Harwood et al., 1999). In Australia, the guidelines have been used in refining estimates of the social costs of drug abuse (alcohol,

The purpose of this appendix is to briefly illustrate the practical application of these guidelines. Since the publication of the first edition of the International Guidelines for Estimating the Costs of Substance Abuse, the guidelines have been used in several COI studies. Among its principal aims, the guidelines are intended to enhance consensus on appropriate methodology and promote greater comparability regarding the results of studies in different countries. By agreement, the authors of the guidelines used the guidelines in subsequent COI studies conducted in Australia, Canada, New Zealand and the U.S. (Collins and Lapsley, 1995; Collins and Lapsley, 1998; Easton, 1998; Single et al., 1998; Harwood et al., 1999).

In Australia the guidelines have been used in refining estimates of the social costs of drug abuse (alcohol, tobacco and illicit drugs) for 1992 (Collins and Lapsley, 1995). They have also been used in estimating the social costs of smoking in these years in two Australian States, Victoria and Western Australia (Collins and Lapsley, 1998). A new study of Australian social costs in the financial year 1998/9, again using the guidelines, is due for completion in the northern Autumn 2002. In Canada a cost estimation study was completed in 1996 utilizing the guidelines (Single et al., 1996; Single et al., 1998). The study is widely cited and used by policy makers and addictions specialists in Canada. A detailed description of data sources was published to assist future updating of the cost estimates (Choi et al., 1997). To address one of many research needs identified by the cost study, the Canadian Centre on Substance Abuse subsequently developed a special research project aimed at providing more exact estimates of the proportion of crime attributable to alcohol and drug use in Canada (Pernanen et al., 2002). The guidelines were similarly the basis for cost estimation studies in New Zealand (Easton, 1997), the U.S. (Harwood et al., 1999) and the Czech Republic (Zabransky et al., 2001). The reader is referred to these studies for examples of how the methods discussed in these guidelines have been applied to generate estimates of the costs of substance abuse.

While not every cost estimation study has made use of them, it is expected that the guidelines will be increasingly utilized in the future as a growing number of countries are considering or have decided to undertake cost estimation studies. The member states of the Inter-American Agency on Narcotic Drugs (CICAD), which includes all countries in the Western Hemisphere, have agreed to regularly monitor economic costs attributable to illicit drug misuse. CICAD is currently developing a training program based on the guidelines for estimating the costs of illicit drugs and it is expected that pilot cost estimation studies will be initiated in the near future. Training seminars have already been conducted in Chile in 1999 sponsored by CICAD, as well as in Colombia in 2000. The guidelines are also being utilized in other parts of the world. For example, the revised guidelines reported in this document, incorporating greater attention to the problems of estimation in developing countries having less adequate data sources, are already being used as the basis for research projects on the social costs of smoking in several South East Asian countries, including Malaysia, Thailand and Cambodia.

One of the primary purposes of this document is to assist researchers dealing with the many issues involved in estimating the economic costs of substance abuse and to thereby promote greater standardisation in methodology and improved comparability of results. It is expected that there will be further refinements as the body of research literature on the costs of substance abuse continues to grow. Thus, these guidelines should be viewed as a work in progress, subject to continual updating and revision as methodological refinements and better information become available.

References

Abel, E.L. (1985) *Dictionary of Alcohol Use and Abuse: Slang, Terms, and Terminology,* Greenwood Press, Connecticut.

Abram, K., Teplin, L. (1990) Drug Disorder, Mental Illness, and Violence. Pp. 222-248 in NIDA Research Monograph Series, Drugs and Violence: Causes, Correlates, and Consequences. Vol. 103. Rockville, MD: National Institute on Drug Abuse.

Armstrong, B. (1990) Morbidity and mortality in Australia: how much is preventable, in McNeill et al. (eds). *A Handbook of Preventative Medicine.* Edward Arnold.

Becker, G., Murphy, K. (1988) A theory of rational addiction. *Journal of Political Economy* 675-700.

Benson, B., Kim, I., Rasmussen, D., Zuehlke, T. (1992). Is property crime caused by drug use or by drug enforcement policy? *Applied Economics* 24: 674-692.

British Journal of Addiction (1991) Editorial, p.86.

Brochu, S. (1995) Estimating the costs of drug-related crime. Paper presented at the 2nd International Symposium on the Social and Economic Costs of Substance Abuse, Montebello, Quebec.

Brunelle, N., Brochu, S. (1995) La prédiction de la délinquance et de la toxicomanie: les risques, les facteurs de risque. 63ième Congrès de l'ACFAS, 24 mai.

Choi, B., Robson,L., Single, E. (1997) Estimating the economic costs of the abuse of tobacco, alcohol and illicit drugs: a review of methodologies and Canadian data sources. *Chronic Diseases in Canada,* 18: 149-165.

Collins, D., Lapsley, H. (1994) Issues and alternatives in the development of a drug abuse estimation model. Paper presented at the First International Symposium on Estimating the Social and Economic Costs of Substance Abuse, Banff, Canada. Ottawa: Canadian Centre on Substance Abuse.

Collins, D., Lapsley, H. (1991) *Estimating the Economic Costs of Drug Abuse in Australia,* Canberra: Commonwealth of Australia, National Campaign Against Drug Abuse Monograph No. 15.

Collins D., Lapsley H. (1995) *Estimating the Economic Costs of Drug Abuse in Australia.* Canberra: Australian Publishing Services.

Collins, D., Lapsley, H. (1998) Estimating and dis-aggregating the social costs of tobacco. In Abedian, I. et al. (Eds). *The Economics of Tobacco Control: Towards an Optimal Policy Mix.* Cape Town: Applied Fiscal Research Centre, University of Cape Town.

Easton, B. (1997) *The Social Costs of Tobacco Use and Alcohol Misuse.* Public Health Monograph No. 2. Wellington, New Zealand: Wellington School of Medicine.

Ellemann-Jensen P. (1991) The social costs of smoking revisited. *British Journal of Addiction* 87: 957-966.

Elnitsky, S., Abernathy, T. (1993) Calgary's needle exchange program: profile of injection drug users. *Can. Journal of Public Health* 84: 177-180.

Fagan, J., Weis, J. G., Cheng, Y. (1990) Delinquency and Substance Use among Inner-City Students. *Journal of Drug Issues,* 20: 351-402.

Grapendaal, M. (1992) Cutting Their Coat According to Their Cloth: Economic Behavior of Amsterdam Opiate Users. *International Journal of the Addictions,* 27(4), 487-501.

Hall, W., Bell, J., Carless, J. (1993) Crime and Drug Use among Applicants for Methadone Maintenance. *Drug and Alcohol Dependence,* 31(2), 123-129.

Hammersley, R., Forsyth, A., Morrison, V., Davies, J. (1989) The Relationship between Crime and Opioid Use. British Journal of Addiction, 84(9), 1029-1043.

Harwood, H. (1994) Analytical principles and issues in making cost-of-illness estimates for substance abuse. Paper presented at the First International Symposium on Estimating the Social and Economic Costs of Substance Abuse, Banff, Canada.

Harwood, H. et al. (1999) *The Economic Costs of Alcohol and Drug Abuse in the United States-1992,* Washington: National Institute on Drug Abuse.

Holman, D. and Armstrong, B. (1990) *The Quantification of Drug Caused Morbidity and Mortality in Australia 1988,* Volumes I and II, Canberra: Department of Community Services and Health.

Hyman, D. (1996) *Public Finance: A Contemporary Application of Theory to Policy.* Fifth edition. London: The Dryden Press.

Jacob, M., Fehr, K. (1987) *The Addiction Research Foundation's Drugs and Drug Abuse: A Reference Text,* Toronto.

Jha, P., Chaloupka, F. (1999) *Curbing the Epidemic. Governments and the Economics of Tobacco Control,* World Bank.

Jha, P., Chaloupka, F. (eds). (2000) *Tobacco control in developing countries,* Oxford University Press.

Kreuzer, A. (1993) Drugs and Delinquency, *EuroCriminology,* 5-6, Lodz.

Lightwood, J., Collins, D., Lapsley, H., Novotny, T. (2000) "Estimating the costs of tobacco use", Chapter 3 of Jha, P., Chaloupka, F. (eds). *Tobacco control in developing countries,* Oxford University Press.

Manning, W., Keeler E., Newhouse J., Sloss E., Wasserman J. (1991) *The Costs of Poor Health Habits.* A RAND Study. Cambridge: Harvard University.

Markandya A., Pearce D. (1989) The social costs of tobacco smoking. *British Journal of Addiction* 84:1139-1150.

Maynard, A., Godfrey C., Hardman, G. (1994) Conceptual issues in estimating the social costs of alcohol. Paper presented at the First International Symposium on Estimating the Social and Economic Costs of Substance Abuse, Banff, Canada. Ottawa: Canadian Centre on Substance Abuse.

McBride, D., McCoy, C. (1981) Crime and drug using behavior. *Criminology,* 19: 281-302.

Millson, P., Myers, T., Rankin, J., McLaughlin, B., Major, C., Mindell, W., Coates, R., Rigby, J., Strathdee, S. (1995) Prevalence of Human Immunodeficiency Virus and associated risk factors in injection drug users in Toronto. *Can. Journal of Public Health* 86: 176-180.

Murray, C., Evans, D., Acharya, A., Baltussen, R. (2000) Development of WHO guidelines on generalized cost-effectiveness analysis. *Health Economics* 9: 235-251.

Murray, C., Lopez, A. (eds). (1996), *The Global Burden of Disease,* Cambridge, Mass.: Harvard University.

Pernanen, K., Cousineau, M.-M., Brochu, S., Sun, F. (2002) Proportions of crimes associated with alcohol and other drugs in Canada. Ottawa: Canadian Centre on Substance Abuse.

Productivity Commission (1990) *Report of the Productivity Commission on Gambling.* Melbourne: Productivity Commission, government of Australia (http://www. Pc.gov.au).

Rice D. (1966) *Estimating the Cost of Illness.* Health Economics Series, no. 6. Rockville, MD: Department of Health, Education and Welfare. DHEW Publication No. (PHS) 947-6.

Rice D. (1993) The economic cost of alcohol abuse and alcohol dependence. *Alcohol Health and Research World* 18:10-11.

Rice D., Hodson T., Kopstein A. (1985) The economic costs of illness: a replication and update. Health Care Financing Review 7:61-80.

Rice D., Hodgson T., Sinsheimer P., Browner W., Kopstein A. (1986) The economic costs of the health effects of smoking, 1984. *The Millbank Quarterly* 64:489-547.

Rice D., Kelman S., Miller L. (1991) Economic costs of drug abuse. (eds). Cartwright WS & Kaple JM. *Economic costs, Cost-effectiveness, Financing and Community-based Drug Treatment.* NIDA Monograph Series No. 113, 10-32.

Rice D., Kelman S., Miller L., Dunmeyer S. (1990) *The Economic Cost of Alcohol and Drug Abuse and Mental Illness 1985.* Report submitted to the Office of Financing and Coverage Policy of the Alcohol, Drug Abuse, and Mental Health Administration. San Francisco: Institute for Health and Aging, University of California. DHHS Publication No. (ADM) 90-1694.

Roth, J. (1994) *Psychoactive Substances and Violence.* Rockville: National Institute of Justice-Research in Brief. Washington: U.S. Department of Justice.

Single E., Collins D., Easton B., Harwood H., Lapsley H., Maynard A. (1996) *International Guidelines on Estimating the Costs of Substance Abuse,* Ottawa: Canadian Centre on Substance Abuse.

Single, E., Robson, L., Rehm, J., Xie, X. (1996) *The Costs of Substance Abuse in Canada,* Ottawa: Canadian Centre on Substance Abuse.

Single, E., Robson, L., Xie, X., Rehm, J. (1998) The economic costs of alcohol, tobacco and illicit drugs in Canada, 1992, *Addiction* 93: 983-998.

Zabranski, T., Mravcik, V., Gajdosikova, H., Miovsky, M. (2001) PAD: Impact Analysis Project of New Drugs Legislation (Final Summary Report). Prague: Office of the Czech Government, Secretariat of the National Drug Commission.

Endnotes

1 The papers presented were: David Collins and Helen Lapsley, "Issues and Alternatives in the Development of a Drug Abuse Estimation Model"; Henrick Harwood, "Analytical Principles and Issues in Making Cost of Illness Estimates for Substance Abuse"; and Alan Maynard, Christine Godfrey and G. Hardman, "Conceptual Issues in Estimating the Social Costs of Alcohol".

2 D.Collins & H.Lapsley, *Estimating the Economic Costs of Drug Abuse in Australia,* National campaign Against Drug Abuse Monograph No.15, 1991.

3 Or Gross National Product (GNP) in the United States.

4 *Theoretical Issues in Abuse Cost Estimation,* paper prepared after the symposium.

5 Even so we ignore the effects of passive smoking, in order to keep the story as simple as possible.

6 Again the concept needs to be treated with care. Implicit in the counterfactual scenario is that the potential production from the greater productivity of the substance abuse is realised or, insofar that it is not, the potential is taken up in voluntary leisure with the same value as the additional production (and not involuntary unemployment).

7 Pressed between the economic and policy logic, and cultural and religious or spiritual sensitivities, participants at the International Symposium on Estimating the Social and Economic Costs of Substance Abuse could not resolve the question of the treatment of the valuation of life. Instead it was suggested to use a deliberately clumsy term of *social gains from additional (quality) life years.* The term "social" is not meant to connote a gain in a religious sense, but to indicate that society may (or may not) value any improvements in the quality of life as a result of reduction in substance abuse. In making this suggestion the proposers were aware they were putting the matter into a temporary limbo, rather than ultimately resolving the philosophical issue. That will depend upon a wider range of professions than even those at the symposium. After that resolution economists can turn to the question of the best valuation method, if any. In the interim a number of methods are advocated, their choice depending on the resolving the deeper philosophical issue.

8 There is another variant of COI studies which might be considered a third approach. Manning and his colleagues (1991), in contrast to the studies by Dorothy Rice (Rice, 1966; Rice et al., 1985; Rice et al., 1986; Rice et al., 1990; Rice et al., 1991; Rice, 1993), strictly limits cost estimates to external costs (paid by others). Furthermore, Manning's external cost approach is incidence-based and utilizes a lifetime model of use. Thus the cost-benefit totals represent the current value of present and future substance use.

9 Assuming that it had done so in the past.

10 Over time the unavoidable costs diminish, so that the CBA counterfactual scenario has a growing stream of cost savings from the smok-

ing cessation. Typically these are *discounted* to give a present value of the avoided costs. Discounting amounts to summing together all those costs, but the further a cost is in the future, the less weight it is given, because it is generally taken that income and spending in the future is less valuable than the same activity in the present. Typically the weighting involves a discount rate, whose magnitude is a matter of contention among economists, although there is widespread agreement that the concept is correct in principle. It follows that not only should the costs of medical care be estimated through time, discounting them to a *present value,* but so should other costs such as productivity and mortality losses.

[11] A common difference is that the treatment the evaluator is looking at, may reduce but not eliminate the illness, so only a proportion of the COI items will be relevant. Sometimes the proportion will differ from item to item.

[12] According to Benson et al. (1992:690), "drug use may cause crime among a subset of about 15 to 25% of the drug-using population but there are other plausible reasons for the apparent correlation between property crime and drug use". A study to determine the aetiologic fraction of property and violent crime that may be causally attributed to illicit drug use is currently underway under the auspices of the Canadian Centre on Substance Abuse.

[13] The anti-drug prevention is often general and then is not a direct concern of the drug budgets. For example, a campaign actualising the healthy life for the youth is not directly labelled "drug" and cannot then be charged to the drug budget. Only the campaigns which directly targeted drug enter the budget. The sums spent in this way are uneasy to calculate and of little importance in the sight of the repression and health expenses.

[14] This approach accordingly does not address the conceptual issues associated with any enjoyment or benefit that consumers derive from use of psychoactive substances. Nor does this approach deal with the fact that resources used to address the problems of psychoactive substances are creating new jobs – actually different jobs, since the funds are taken away from other uses that would themselves create jobs. Also, the theoretical economic constructs of "consumer's surplus", marginal utility analysis, and social welfare functions are beyond the scope of this analysis.

[15] *System of National Accounts:* 1993, published by Commission of the European Communities (Union), International Bank for Reconstruction and Development ("World Bank"). International Monetary Fund, Organization for Economic Cooperation and Development, and the United Nations.

[16] Because the SNA framework involves a set of subsidiary tables – the most important for these purposes are the household, public, producer, and (perhaps) rest-of-world sectors – it may be useful to split the COI estimate into these components. It makes sense to separate out an account for the drug users from the household account, and it will be as useful to separate the production activities of the drug suppliers out from the producer account. Fully elaborated, there will be interaction between the subsidiary tables, as when the taxes paid by the user (if any) will be payments in the private user account, and a receipt in the public sector account. Ideally the accounts could be set out so their net balance is equal to the COI.

[17] This glossary was written by Brian Easton and Robert Bowie for the first edition of these guidelines, with some additional terms drafted by Eric Single. The authors are grateful to David Collins and Helen Lapsley for a comment on an earlier draft, but take full responsibility for any errors and omissions.